An Ageless Woman's Guide to Heart Health

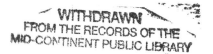

Your path to lifelong wellness

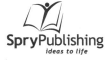
Elizabeth Jackson, MD, MPH

SpryPublishing
ideas to life

This edition is published by Spry Publishing LLC
2500 South State Street
Ann Arbor, MI 48104 USA

Printed and bound in the United States of America.

10 9 8 7 6 5 4 3 2 1

Library of Congress Control Number: 2013933246
Paperback ISBN: 978-1-938170-22-5
E-book ISBN: 978-1-938170-23-2

Disclaimer: Spry Publishing LLC does not assume responsibility
for the contents or opinions expressed herein. Although every precaution is
taken to ensure that information is accurate as of the date of publication,
differences of opinion exist. The opinions expressed herein are those of the
author and do not necessarily reflect the views of the publisher. The
information contained in this book is not intended to replace professional
advisement of an individual's doctor prior to beginning or
changing an individual's course of treatment.

To the lights of my life—Anders and Aric

With Every Beat

INTRODUCTION

The best and most beautiful things in the world cannot be seen or even touched—they must be felt with the heart.

HELEN KELLER

Have you ever been told that you have a "good heart"? Or perhaps you "wear your heart on your sleeve." The heart has long been symbolic of kindness, generosity, and love. Just think of all those heart-shaped boxes of chocolate given on Valentine's Day! When we fall in love, our hearts sometimes skip a beat, and when we witness our children's accomplishments our hearts swell with pride. If we want to find true happiness, we are often told to follow our hearts. Women in particular are often described as the "heart of the home." As a woman and mother of two teenage boys, I couldn't agree more. But, as a cardiologist with over 20 years of experience in health care, I also have a more clinical view of the heart.

To me, having a good heart means not only that you are kind, but that your heart muscle is strong and healthy! This remarkable muscular pump beats approximately 100,000 times each day, circulating 2,000 gallons of blood through our bodies. Over a normal life span, the heart will beat more than 2.5 billion times. Our hearts assist our lungs, our kidneys, and our digestive system and provide our cells, muscles, and brain with necessary nourishment. In short, we cannot live without our hearts. Maybe that's why the heart has become synonymous with such strong, positive emotions.

Unfortunately, this vital, hardworking muscle has a formidable enemy: heart disease. *Heart disease is the leading cause of death for both men and women.* In fact, though women tend to fear cancer the most, heart disease is actually the leading cause of death among women of all ages. Today, more than 6.5 million American women suffer from coronary heart disease, and since 1984, more American women than men have died from heart disease. Are you surprised?

Heart disease has long been thought of as a men's issue, but as you can see from the statistics, it's an equal-opportunity health problem. What is happening? Are more women getting heart disease than before? No, women have always been at risk; it's just that scientific research regarding that risk is relatively new. During the first 80 years or so of the twentieth century, the medical community was made up of predominantly male doctors, who studied and treated heart disease in men. They believed that estrogen protected women from the plaque buildup that occurs in blood vessels and leads to cardiovascular problems. Although estrogen does provide some protection up to a certain age (which we will discuss later in the book), other risk factors are just as prevalent in women as men. New research, involving women, has shed much-needed light on this important issue.

We have learned that heart disease often affects women differently from men. And yet, there are more similarities than differences. Family history, high cholesterol, high blood pressure, diabetes, smoking, and lifestyle issues are the risk factors associated with heart disease for men and women. In both cases, prevention is the best treatment! When it comes to heart disease, changing your lifestyle can save your life.

That's the first reason I decided to write this book. Although awareness regarding women and heart disease has increased (e.g., the Red Dress Campaign) and information is more readily available than ever before, we still have a long way to go. As they say, knowledge is power; if you understand how the heart works, what keeps it functioning properly, how to avoid risk factors, and what warning signs and symptoms to look for, you can save your life—or the life of a loved one. That's powerful stuff.

Secondly, if women are truly the heart of the home, and I believe in many cases they are, you can make a huge difference in your family's health. Despite societal changes, women are, for the most part, still primarily responsible for grocery shopping and meal preparation. We are typically the ones who make doctor's appointments, urge spouses and children to get medical treatment, and care for elderly parents. As *mothers, the decisions we make every day can go a long way toward instilling heart-healthy habits in our children—habits that will serve them well for life. By becoming better educated on heart disease, you can have a positive impact on the people in your life.*

While we often do a great job caring for our families and others, women tend to ignore their own health issues, and that is the third reason for this endeavor. Every day, I see patients with cardiovascular concerns, from the routine to the life-threatening. I typically spend more time talking to my patients than actually examining them. I find that listening to people gives me a more complete picture of their health—and what a patient tells me can be just as enlightening as an EKG. During these conversations, I have found that women have a tendency to focus more on others and, as a result, put off seeing a physician about their own health until things become serious. They are often able to recite their spouse's cholesterol level or blood pressure more readily than their own.

I want that to change. I want you to take care of yourself, and know your numbers—cholesterol, blood pressure, sugar—and what those numbers mean. I want you to understand your risk factors and what to do about them. I want you to be aware of the early warning signs of a heart attack and not wait until it's too late to be treated. I want you to be a role model for your family and friends. If I could, I would sit down and talk to every woman in the world about the importance of heart health, but since that's impossible, this book is the next best thing.

If the information on these pages motivates you to eat healthier and exercise more; if it prompts you to know your risk factors and begin a dialogue with your health-care provider; even if it simply nudges you into taking one small step toward heart health, I will have accomplished my goal. Why, just thinking about it fills my heart with joy!

It's Never Too Late

You may have picked up this book because you or someone you love is already dealing with cardiovascular problems. Or maybe you have a family history of heart disease and want to take steps to reduce your own risk. Perhaps you are just curious about all the news related to heart disease in women these days. Whether you are healthy and seeking guidelines for prevention or have already experienced a heart attack and wish to regain control of your health, I think you'll find the information helpful. One thing I have learned over the years, in both my personal and professional life, is that it's never too late to make a positive change.

My life plan did not initially include becoming a cardiologist. Though I found science interesting in high school and college, it wasn't my favorite subject. In fact, I majored in art and art history! While considering art conservation as a possible career, I discovered that one needed a basic understanding of chemistry, which I found intriguing. This interest, coupled with a strong desire to help others, led me to start working in a cardiologist's office. The nurses, technicians, doctors, and patients at that office opened up a whole new world for me. The more I learned about the heart, the more I wanted to know.

Before I knew it, I had a job performing electrocardiograms in a Boston hospital and was taking premedical courses at night. It took five long years of working during the day and going to school in the evenings, but I finally achieved my dream of attending medical school. Along the way, my interest in cardiology continued to grow. Now, as a cardiologist at one of the most-respected medical facilities in the country, I find that my initial awe at the way our hearts function has not waned. Each day, I continue to learn more and gain new appreciation for this amazing organ system.

I understand that life can take you in many directions. Like my career path, your journey toward heart health may not be easy or straightforward; it may be filled with detours and setbacks. However, as long as you continue forward, making positive changes—no matter how small—you can improve your health. With that in mind, I have included simple *steps you can take to protect and improve your heart health at the end of every chapter. So, no matter where you are in your journey—younger or older, healthy or ailing—I hope you'll take this book along as your guide. May it inspire you to take good care of yourself and provide the support you need to lead a heart-healthy life.*

ELIZABETH JACKSON

CHAPTER ONE

With Every Beat

Wherever you go, go with all your heart.

CONFUCIUS

Your heart beats approximately 100,000 times each day. Whether you are busy at work, out running a marathon, or relaxing on the couch, your heart is adjusting to the changing demands of your body, pumping thousands of gallons of blood through your veins and arteries, also known as your circulatory system. In a healthy circulatory system, all this happens without your giving it much thought. In fact, until something goes wrong—we experience chest pain or breathlessness, for instance—most people don't think about their hearts and how these amazing organs function. So, before we discuss what keeps a heart healthy or what can cause it to malfunction, it's helpful to have a basic understanding of the heart's structure and how it works.

The Structure and Function of the Heart

Located in the upper left chest, next to the lungs, the heart has a very simple main function—to pump blood. The heart is a fist-sized muscle that works like other muscles in your body; that is, the muscle cells contract to get the job done. When you lift a child in your arms or use your legs to run, the heart is continuously contracting and pumping blood throughout your body.

But let's start at the very beginning. In the first several weeks after conception, groups of cells that will become the heart are forming. The initial structure looks like a tube. In a truly awe-inspiring feat, this tube twists and turns and eventually is transformed into a complex organ. When fully developed, the heart has four chambers with two *atria* (located at the top) and two *ventricles* (located at the bottom). Between these chambers are doorways, called heart valves.

The heart starts to beat soon after conception—about 21 days or five weeks after a woman's last period. The heart begins this process by taking deoxygenated blood (i.e., blood that's been depleted of oxygen by our other organs) returning through veins into the right atrium and ventricle. This deoxygenated blood enters the heart through two large veins called the *vena cava*. The chambers on the right side of the heart funnel the blood into the arteries in the lungs, where the red blood cells receive oxygen. The oxygenated blood then returns from the lungs into the left side of the heart, first into the left atrium and then into the left ventricle. The left ventricle, which is the main pumping chamber, forcefully contracts and pumps the blood out to the arteries, which bring oxygen-rich blood to the rest of the body, including your muscles and your brain. Without the heart's contractions, other organs in our bodies cannot function. Every heartbeat is truly life-sustaining, and without heartbeats death occurs. Fortunately for us, the heart is an involuntary muscle, unlike our leg and arm muscles, which are under our control. The heart pumps without our thinking about it.

That's a basic overview of how the heart functions. If we look more closely, we can see that the process is bit more complex. Figure 1 shows the route our blood takes entering and leaving the heart. The journey goes like this:

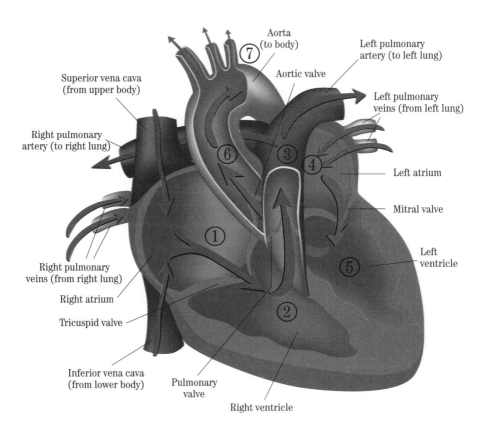

Figure 1. Cross-section diagram of the heart with blood flow.

- The first stop for blood returning to our hearts through our veins is the right atrium (1). This is also where the heartbeat starts. A group of cells known as the pacemaker cells, which are located in the upper right atrium, start the contraction of the upper heart. Your heartbeat, calculated as beats per minute, is controlled by this area of the heart. When you run to catch a bus, for instance, the increase in your heart rate is initiated here. There is a second area of pacemaker cells closer to the ventricle, but also located in the right atrium, that help regulate our heart rates. If we experience problems with the heart's rhythm, such as heart palpitations or a racing heartbeat, this is the area to which we focus our attention.
- If you think of the chambers of the heart as separate rooms, then the doors between those rooms are the valves. Unlike the doors in our houses, however, these doors should open only one way. When the right ventricle (2) contracts, the valve between the right atrium and the right ventricle stays shut so that blood does not go backward. In other words, the valves keep the blood flowing in one direction. When people have very high blood pressure in their lungs or the right ventricle cannot pump effectively, the valve between the right atrium and ventricle does not work well, and blood backs up in the veins. If this happens, patients often have swelling in their lower extremities and abdomen.
- When the blood enters the right ventricle, it's pumped from the ventricle to the lungs (3). Again, the valve that sits between the right ventricle and the lungs makes sure the blood only goes one way—forward into the lungs, where it receives oxygen. After the blood receives oxygen from the lungs, it travels back to the heart and into the left atrium (4), where it is pumped into the left ventricle (5) through another one-way

valve. As mentioned earlier, the left side of the heart is the main pumping chamber. When heart attacks or heart failure occurs, the majority of problems are located in the left system. For instance, when the left ventricle does not pump effectively the blood can back up into the lungs, making breathing more difficult. Sometimes the valves on the left side of the heart do not open or close normally, which can also cause problems with blood being pumped forward. When blood moves backward, we call this *heart failure*. (We'll take a closer look at some of these potential problems in chapter 2.)

> The circulatory or vascular system consists of the heart, the lungs, and all the blood vessels (veins and arteries) that form a network through our bodies. If these vessels were laid end to end, they would be approximately 100,000 miles long! The heart pumps 2,000 gallons of blood through these vessels every day to deliver essential oxygen and nutrients throughout the body and to remove carbon dioxide and other cellular waste products.

- After blood leaves the heart it travels through the *aorta* (6), which is the largest artery in the body. There are three major coronary arteries that branch out from the aorta. These are very important arteries because they carry oxygenated blood directly to the heart muscle. Most heart disease is caused by problems with these arteries. When blockages from *atherosclerosis* or hardening of the arteries occur in these vessels, it makes it difficult for the heart to receive oxygen, which may cause chest pain and sometimes a heart attack. We will discuss coronary arteries and their related problems, including how arterial disease in women may differ from the disease men experience, in much more detail later in the book.

- Finally, like a protective layer of bubble wrap, there is tissue around the heart called the *pericardium*. Between the heart and the pericardium is a small amount of fluid that allows the heart to be gently cushioned in the pericardial sac. Occasionally this sac can become inflamed and cause chest pain, a condition referred to as *pericarditis*. In addition, the sac may sometimes have more fluid than normal, making it more difficult for the heart to beat.

- Connecting your heart to the rest of the body are blood vessels called veins and arteries. You can think of veins and arteries as a network of one-way streets. As a cardiologist, I am just as concerned with the condition of these "streets" as with the heart itself. Veins work to bring deoxygenated blood back to your heart, while arteries carry oxygen-rich blood out of the heart and throughout your body. In the same way a traffic jam can cause major chaos on the roadways, clogged veins and arteries can lead to big problems with your heart, as well as other areas of the body. And, as we learned earlier, one of the main highways or arteries in your body is the aorta.

- The aorta starts at the left ventricle and then arches through your chest and down into your trunk (7). It has many branches, which travel up to your brain and down your arms and legs. Keeping the aorta and other arteries free of atherosclerosis,

An Ounce of Prevention

We know more about the structure and function of the heart, as well as what causes it to malfunction, than ever before. Over the past several decades, significant progress has been made regarding the diagnosis and treatment of cardiovascular diseases. Yet heart disease is still the leading cause of death for both men and women in the United States. Even with today's availability of highly effective medications, the best treatment for heart disease is prevention.

which is essentially a buildup of plaque, is a key component of heart health. Because the heart is part of the vascular or circulatory system, problems that affect the vascular system often stem from the same risk factors that are associated with heart disease, including hypertension (high blood pressure), smoking, high cholesterol, or diabetes.

Take a Step

You've already taken an important first step toward heart health. By learning how the heart functions and the important role veins and arteries play in keeping the heart pumping effectively, circulating blood throughout our bodies, you're better able to understand what can go wrong and what you can do about it. Your next step is to learn more about potential problems with the heart, including the number-one killer of both men and women—heart disease, along with the warning signs and symptoms of a heart attack.

CHAPTER TWO

Heart Problems

A good head and good heart are always a formidable combination.

NELSON MANDELA

Having a good heart is important, but having a strong, healthy heart is absolutely essential. Think of the heart as the motor or pump in a complex system. The system cannot run without a motor. When you consider how hard our hearts work—24 hours a day, every day—and how little maintenance they require, it's remarkable. However, as with any intricate piece of machinery with many parts, there are numerous things that can go wrong.

Potential Problems with the Heart

Congenital Defects Some heart problems occur prior to birth, as the heart is developing. These congenital defects are much less common than heart attacks or strokes and can be quite complex. Given the limitations of this book, we will not discuss congenital heart defects in detail. Please refer to the American Heart Association (AHA) web site, www.heart.org/, for more information.

Arrhythmias Our heartbeats are controlled by electrical impulses that coordinate the beats. When there are problems with the heart's electrical or rhythm system, we experience abnormal or irregular heartbeats called arrhythmias. Arrhythmias can cause the heart to beat too fast, too slow, or erratically. They are fairly common, especially among women. In fact, the majority of people will experience an occasional fluttering or racing heartbeat during their lives. Most of these arrhythmias are completely harmless, but some can be deadly. For instance, if the disturbance in the heart's rhythm is so severe that the heart can no longer beat in a way that pumps blood to the rest of the body, death can occur within minutes. That's why you'll find a growing number of automatic external defibrillators (AEDs) in public areas. A shock from an AED can potentially restore a proper heart rhythm. We will discuss heart rhythms in much more detail in the following chapter.

Valves As we saw in chapter 1, the valves between the chambers of our hearts act as one-way doors, making sure blood flows in only one direction. Sometimes the heart valves can start to function abnormally, allowing blood to back up and not flow properly through the chambers. This condition is sometimes referred to as leaking valves (or regurgitation). Valves may also become narrow, often due to calcification, though this is rare. Valve problems are more likely to occur as we age.

Heart Failure This is a fairly common problem, especially among the elderly—and particularly among women. It occurs when the heart muscle becomes too weak to pump enough blood to meet the body's demands. The weakness is most often the result of heart attacks, which damage or kill heart cells. However, cardiovascular disease, high blood pressure, and diabetes can also lead to heart failure. This condition may affect either side of the heart, and sometimes both. When the right side of the heart is weak, the heart can't pump enough blood to the lungs to pick up oxygen, causing fluid to build up in the feet, ankles, legs, liver, abdomen, and veins of the neck. Left-sided heart failure occurs when the heart is unable to pump enough oxygen-rich blood to the rest of the body, causing fluid to accumulate in the lungs, shortness of breath, and extreme fatigue. You may have also heard the term *congestive heart failure*, which refers to the backup of fluid causing congestion in other parts of our body as the heart fails to pump effectively.

Another type of heart failure may occur when the heart muscle becomes stiff, usually a result of years of hypertension when the heart has to work hard against higher blood pressure. Remember, the heart is a muscle, so when heart muscles work too hard, they can get bigger. This is good for muscles in your legs and arms, but not for your heart. An enlarged heart muscle can become stiff and unable to pump effectively. This can also result in fluid in the lungs, and thus heart failure. It is very common for older women to have high blood pressure, and therefore the number of women with heart failure due to an inefficient heart muscle is significant. As the population ages, it is likely that the number of women experiencing heart failure will also grow.

Atherosclerosis Atherosclerosis, or hardening of the arteries, is a lifelong process that involves the buildup of plaque and thickening of artery walls. It can lead to many diseases, including heart disease. In fact, although there are many problems that can occur in the cardiovascular system, **damage to the heart muscle due to atherosclerosis is the leading cause of heart disease.** But it doesn't have to be.

Just as a piece of machinery, such as a car, requires regular maintenance to keep it running smoothly, our hearts and blood vessels also need proper upkeep. When I think of the amount of

SARA'S STORY

In many ways, Sara is a typical middle-aged woman. At 54, she works full-time as an accountant, and though her children are grown, she is busy caring for her elderly parents. Between her job and her caretaking responsibilities, she has little time for herself. Because time is short, Sara and her husband often rely on quick pasta dishes or takeout for dinner. She does not exercise regularly, but she feels her lifestyle keeps her active—she does most of the household chores and runs errands for both her family and her parents. To relax, Sara smokes three or four cigarettes a day. She has been trying to quit for years but reasons that she is better off smoking just "a couple of cigarettes" rather than an entire pack, which she did during her 30s.

Overall, Sara felt until recently that she was in good health. But one morning, she woke up feeling slightly nauseous. While she was getting ready for work, this nausea increased, but she chalked it up to something she ate or possibly the flu. Unconcerned, Sara drove to work and started in on her daily routine. As the morning progressed, she felt generally ill—the nausea became worse, and she experienced some sweating. When her jaw began to ache, she mentioned it to a coworker, who became concerned. Her coworker told Sara that her husband had had jaw pain during his heart attack. Still, Sara did not believe there was a problem with her heart until she began to feel pressure in her chest—not a crushing pain, but a sensation of heaviness.

At this point she realized she should go to the hospital, and her coworkers called 911. When the emergency medical technicians (EMTs) arrived, they performed an electrocardio-gram (EKG) and notified the hospital that Sara was indeed having a heart attack. The coronary team was alerted, and the cardiac catheterization lab (cath lab) was made ready for her arrival. At the hospital, Sara went directly to the cath lab, where she underwent a coronary angiogram. This test showed a blockage in her right coronary artery. The artery was opened up right away, and a stent was placed in the blocked vessel to keep that area open. Sara was then trans-ferred to the coronary care unit for monitoring.

Two days later, Sara was discharged from the hospital. She had experienced a significant heart attack, and her heart muscle in the area of the attack was permanently damaged, never regaining full function. If she had gone to the hospital sooner, she might have incurred less damage to her heart muscle. She was given medications to protect her from future heart attacks. Sara also went to cardiac rehab for several months after her discharge, which aided tremendously in her recovery. Not only did the rehab program help her develop a regular exercise routine and educate her on the importance of a heart-healthy diet, it encouraged her to finally quit smok-ing.

Though Sara had a heart attack, she is a success story be-cause she adopted and maintained heart-healthy habits, prov-ing that it's never too late to improve your health. One year after her cardiac event, Sara was still not smoking. She had lost ten pounds and was exercising regularly. She continued to take her cardiac medications each day and had no further symptoms. Best of all, Sara told her doctor that she had much more energy than she had had prior to her heart attack.

work a heart has to do throughout one's life, I want to treat mine with extra special care. That doesn't mean you should be a couch potato and not give your heart a workout. On the contrary, regular exercise is essential for your heart. Your heart also needs good fuel in the form of a healthy diet to keep it in prime condition. By taking care of your heart, you will keep it strong, allowing it to pump with vigor throughout your life.

What *Exactly* Is Heart Disease?

Rates of death due to heart disease have declined over the past decade, which is very encouraging. Much of this decline is thought to be due to reductions in risk factors such as smoking. However, we have a long way to go, given that heart disease remains the number-one killer of women (and men). In fact, heart disease and stroke, which are referred to as cardiovascular diseases (CVDs), kill more women than all cancers combined (including breast cancer).

According to the American Heart Association

- From 1998 to 2008, death rates due to cardiovascular disease (CVD) have declined 30.6 percent.
- CVD still accounts for 32.8 percent of all deaths in the United States, or 1 out of every 3 deaths.
- 2,200 Americans die each day from CVD (1 every 39 seconds).
- 1 of every 6 deaths is due to CVD. In 2008, that accounted for 405,309 deaths.
- The annual rate of new coronary events is 785,000, and the rate of recurrent events is approximately 470,000.
- Heart events (mostly heart attacks) occur approximately every 25 seconds. Every minute one American dies from a heart event.

Source: Go AS et al. on behalf of the American Heart Association Statistics Committee and Stroke Statistics Subcommittee. Heart disease and stroke statistics—2013 update: a report from the American Heart Association. *Circulation* 2013.

Any disorder that causes the heart to malfunction is heart disease. However, as mentioned earlier, atherosclerosis is the primary cause of coronary artery disease (CAD), which is what most people are referring to when they talk about heart disease. Since the function of the heart is to keep blood circulating continuously through our vessels, you can see how atherosclerosis can cause major problems with our hearts and circulatory systems.

As we've learned, atherosclerosis involves the thickening and hardening of the walls of our arteries. This thickening comes from a buildup of plaque, which is made up of various fats that are deposited in and adhere to the walls of blood vessels (see Figure 2). The plaque buildup causes the vessels to narrow and restricts proper blood flow. As the vessels become more and more constricted, the heart has to work harder and harder to pump blood through the body, and eventually there is not enough blood to meet the body's demands.

What Causes Plaque?

So, where does this plaque that forms in our arteries come from? There are several sources. First, certain types of cholesterol deposit fat along blood vessels that turns into plaque, while other types of cholesterol (often referred to as good cholesterol) can actually carry plaque away (see chapter 7 for more about the role cholesterol plays in heart health). CVD risk factors such as hypertension (high blood pressure) and diabetes increase the probability of having plaque buildup on the artery walls. Hypertension also causes blood vessels to thicken as they continually fight against the higher blood pressure, further narrowing the arteries. In addition, there are a number of elements, such as genes, gender, smoking, exercise, stress, and obesity that can affect plaque growth and blood vessel

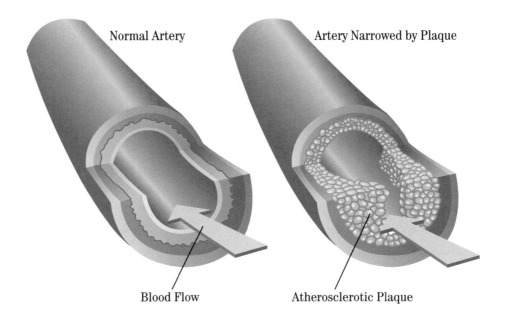

Normal Artery   Artery Narrowed by Plaque

Blood Flow   Atherosclerotic Plaque

Figure 2. Diagram of a normal artery and an artery with narrowing caused by plaque. Plaque buildup narrows the vessels and restricts proper blood flow.

size. For example, increased weight and lack of exercise (and even depression) can increase inflammation in the body and cause vessels to not function properly. We call this *endothelial dysfunction*, and this condition makes it more likely that fat will be deposited into the arteries, which is how plaque builds.

What Is a Heart Attack?

While other things may cause a heart attack, atherosclerosis is the most common culprit. Plaque may be unstable and rupture, causing a heart attack, or build up over time, causing chest pain during activities such as walking. Either way, atherosclerotic plaque is the underlying cause of nearly 75 percent of all cardiovascular deaths. When the plaque in a blood vessel blocks blood flow, and therefore oxygen, to the heart, a heart attack occurs. The most common form of heart disease is a heart attack, also known as a *myocardial infarction*.

The heart muscle needs oxygen to survive. Without oxygen, even for a short period of time, muscle cells start to die. This is what doctors mean when they say "time is muscle." The quicker you get to a hospital and get treated, the less heart muscle will die.

Plaque takes time to develop, and unfortunately it often starts to accumulate in childhood. When the coronary arteries of young men and women are examined, we often find small amounts of plaque already beginning to form. Over time, this plaque not only builds, but can become unstable and cause a sudden heart attack. In simple terms, unstable plaque breaks apart, and our body reacts to this by forming a clot (see Figure 3). Clots are great when you have a cut on your skin; they stop the bleeding. However, in the coronary artery they block blood from flowing to the remainder of the artery. No blood means a lack of oxygen, and the muscle fed by that artery suddenly has no nourishment and will die shortly if blood flow is not returned. We don't know when unstable plaque will break open, which is scary for both patients and their doctors. It would be nice to be able to predict that type of heart attack and prevent it from occurring, but since we can't, it's very important to know the warning signs of a heart attack (see page 33).

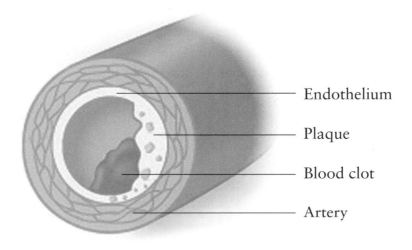

Endothelium

Plaque

Blood clot

Artery

Figure 3. Diseased artery with plaque. Plaque buildup can become unstable and break apart. The body reacts by forming a clot.

Of course, knowing your risk factors and managing them, including leading a heart-healthy lifestyle (i.e., healthy diet, exercise, and stress reduction) can go a long way toward reducing plaque and the likelihood it will become unstable in the first place. Also, for patients who have had a heart attack, certain medications may help prevent another event by reducing plaque and clotting.

What Is Angina?

When we or someone we know experience chest pain, our first thought is typically of a heart attack. In reality, many things may cause chest pain, including indigestion, gallbladder attacks, problems with the esophagus, and angina, to name a few. Angina, which literally means "squeezing of the chest" in Latin, is closely related to heart attack, as it's caused by decreased blood flow and oxygen to the heart muscle. Just as with a heart attack, the reduced blood flow is most often a result of a narrowing of the coronary artery due to atherosclerosis, and the symptoms are very similar.

Angina can be described as pressure, heaviness, tightening, squeezing, or aching across the chest, particularly behind the breastbone. The pain can sometimes radiate to the neck, jaw, arms, back, or even teeth. However, unlike a heart attack, the supply of blood and oxygen to the heart is not completely cut off, and the condition can cause chronic chest pain.

There are two types of angina: stable and unstable. Stable angina is the most common and is what most people mean when they refer to angina. Patients with stable angina have symptoms on a regular basis; for instance, walking up the stairs always causes chest pain. Exertion is typically the trigger for stable angina, although severe emotional stress or a heavy meal can also bring it on—anything that causes the heart to demand more blood oxygen than the arteries can supply. The discomfort usually lasts from 1 to 15 minutes and is relieved by resting or placing a nitroglycerin tablet under the tongue. Nitroglycerin relaxes the blood vessels and lowers blood pressure, which improves blood flow.

Unstable angina is less common, but more serious. The symptoms are more severe and less predictable than stable angina. In addition, the pain is often more frequent, lasts longer, occurs at rest, and may not be relieved by nitroglycerin. While unstable angina is not the same as a heart attack, it warrants an immediate visit to your health-care provider or emergency room for further cardiac testing. This condition is often a precursor to a heart attack.

Warning Signs of a Heart Attack

A heart attack is serious business. Many people do not recognize the signs of a heart attack and, therefore, do not get to the hospital in a timely manner. Unfortunately, a delay might mean that someone never makes it to the hospital. Over half of all coronary events end in sudden death. Delaying treatment may also cause more damage to the heart. In other words, time is muscle. The sooner treatment is started, the more likely someone will prevent significant damage to his or her heart.

The range of symptoms experienced during a heart attack can vary widely, from nothing at all to death. The warning signs someone may feel depends on which heart cells are not receiving oxygen and how severe the deprivation is. Typically, when heart cells begin to die, people experience chest pain. This doesn't mean that all chest pain indicates a heart attack, or that everyone who experiences a heart attack will have chest pain. However, chest pain is still the most common symptom of a heart attack.

Classic warning signs of a heart attack include chest pain or chest pressure, which may first occur with exercise or exertion, or even the stress of strong emotions. Sometimes this discomfort spreads to the arms (particularly the left arm) and/or jaw. Many people also relate a feeling of weakness and experience sweating and nausea, which sometimes leads to vomiting. Others may have problems breathing. When chest pressure or pain occurs at rest, or does not go away with rest, this is a particularly worrisome sign.

After reviewing 69 studies, investigators from one larger analysis found that women report having no chest pain at the time of a coronary event more often than men. However, the majority of women (63–70 percent) did report chest pain. (Canto et al., *Arch Intern Med*. 2007;167(22): 2405–2411.)

For women, it may be more difficult to recognize the signs of a heart attack, since we often have symptoms that are not considered classic. That doesn't mean, however, that chest pain or pressure is uncommon among women. Several studies show that women have chest pain at similar rates to men. On the flip side, many other studies have noted that women may experience atypical symptoms, with or without chest pain, including:

- unusual levels of fatigue in the days or weeks before an attack
- shortness of breath, which may begin days or even weeks preceding the attack. Many women report gasping or having trouble talking.
- nausea or upset stomach, and sometimes dizziness (feeling as though you may faint)
- heavy sweating for no apparent reason, or feeling both hot and chilled, with clammy skin
- pain or pressure in other areas of the body, such as the neck, jaw, shoulders or upper back. This can include general soreness or achiness, rather than the "crushing" pain often associated with heart attacks.
- anxiety or the feeling of impending doom (call it women's intuition)

For a more detailed explanation of these warning signs, please see chapter 4.

Now, I know many of you zeroed in on the first symptom, "fatigue," and are probably thinking, "I'm always tired. Does that mean I have a heart problem?" Probably not—most women feel fatigued at some point! The key word here is "unusual." If you are suddenly feeling extremely fatigued, and this is a new symptom, that warrants concern.

For both women and men, here are some of the general

warning signs of a heart attack (from The American Heart Association, www.goredforwomen.org/about_heart_disease_and_stroke.aspx)

- chest pain or pressure (sometimes described as a squeezing)
- pain, discomfort, or numbness in the arms, back, jaw, or stomach
- shortness of breath
- a cold sweat, nausea, or light-headedness

Treatment for a Heart Attack

The most important factor in the treatment of a heart attack is restoring blood flow to the heart muscle, which is oxygen starved. That's why it's critical for women to recognize the signs and symptoms of an acute coronary event and not hesitate to seek treatment. Remember, if too many heart cells are damaged, the heart may no longer pump effectively, which can lead to heart failure.

Typical treatment for a heart attack may include:

- **An electrocardiogram (EKG)**—Once the emergency team is alerted, an EKG is the first step in helping to determine the type of heart attack someone is experiencing. EKGs are so important that many areas of the country have put special initiatives in place to make sure EKGs are completed in the field. In other words, the emergency response team that takes you to the hospital are the ones who initiate the first steps of treatment, including taking an EKG and transmitting it to the emergency room physician and the cardiologist. For this reason, it's very important to call 911 rather than have someone else drive you to the hospital.

- **Aspirin and other medications**—The emergency team will usually administer a dose of aspirin (often four children's aspirins—or 81 mg × 4). Aspirin helps prevent platelets (the cells in our blood that help it clot) from adhering together, therefore improving blood flow. It's usually the first of several medications that patients receive during the treatment of a heart attack. If you are allergic to aspirin, let your health-care providers (including the emergency response team) know right away. There are other medications available. Once in the hospital, most patients receive additional medications like heparin or a similar drug to prevent further clotting, as well as medication to lower blood pressure and help the heart pump efficiently. The American Heart Association and the American College of Cardiology have online information on the majority of medications and treatment you may receive in the course of a hospitalstay for an acute coronary syndrome. Visit www.heart.org and search "treatment of heart attack."
- **Cardiac catheterization**—Many patients will also visit the cardiac catheterization lab, where a long, thin, flexible tube called a catheter is inserted into a blood vessel in the arm, groin, or neck and threaded to the heart. Through the catheter, a doctor can do diagnostic tests and, in some cases, perform treatments on the heart. For example, the catheter may be filled with a special dye that flows through your bloodstream to the heart. As the dye flows through the blood vessels, a series of X-ray images of the coronary arteries is taken. This procedure is called a *coronary angiogram*.

If the catheter locates a blockage that can be opened, the cardiologist will perform a percutaneous coronary intervention (PCI). A PCI opens the blocked artery by first placing a balloon in the area that is blocked. The balloon is then inflated to expand the narrowing caused by the plaque and open the artery wider. Stents are often placed in the narrow section to further widen the vessel and keep it open. A PCI is often a lifesaving procedure, particularly for certain types of heart attacks. In some cases, such as with unstable angina, patients may not need to go immediately to the catheterization lab; and those who are at very low risk may do just as well with medications.

What if a patient is too far away from a hospital that can perform a PCI? If a catheterization lab is not readily available, specialized medications can help break up the blockage and increase blood flow to the heart until further treatment is available.

- **Bypass surgery**—For some patients, the extent of the blockage makes PCI ineffective, and coronary artery bypass graft surgery (CABG) is recommended. This type of open-heart surgery uses veins (often from the legs) and sometimes arteries to route blood around the blockages. CABG is a significant surgery, often requiring the sternum (or breast-bone) to be cut open for better access to the heart. The heart is then stopped from beating, and the patient's blood is circulated and oxygenated in a special machine while the surgeons complete the bypass procedure. The patient will then need to recover for several days in the hospital, followed by additional recuperative time at home or in a special rehabilitation facility.

Cardiac Rehabilitation

After being discharged from the hospital, women who have experienced a cardiac event should ask their doctors about enrolling in a cardiac rehabilitation program. **It's a well-known fact that women do not enter or complete these programs as often as men.** There are several reasons why this may be happening. First, younger women are frequently balancing family and work obligations and are therefore reluctant to take the time to complete a rehab program. For older women, the issue is typically related to access. They are less likely to be able to drive and hesitant to ask family or friends to take them. Since women are usually older at the time of a heart attack, and may have other illnesses or mobility issues, some doctors may assume these patients are not interested in this type of program. However, even if a woman has difficulty walking, she can complete a cardiac rehab program and benefit tremendously. **Data show that these programs greatly reduce mortality after a coronary event.**

Cardiac rehabilitation is a structured program that often starts in the hospital with education about having a heart attack and the treatment plan, which is referred to as phase one. Phase two occurs as an outpatient, when the heart attack survivor visits a rehab facility several times per week over the course of several months. Recently, Medicare increased coverage for the number of weeks a patient is eligible for cardiac rehabilitation, based on the benefits gained from such programs.

Cardiac rehab provides an evaluation of your cardiac and medical history, along with your baseline fitness. An exercise program is then tailored to you, and sessions are performed under the supervision of trained staff—with heart rate and blood pressure monitoring. Most programs also offer education and counseling on diet, stress, and smoking cessation. Participants learn to set reasonable goals, based on their individual condition, in order to achieve a heart-healthy lifestyle.

After phase two is completed, many programs offer the option to continue to exercise at the cardiac rehabilitation facilities, which is called phase three. During this phase, participants are not monitored as closely, but they do have the benefit of interacting with trained personnel who have come to know them. This can help patients stick to the program.

Cardiac rehabilitation programs are also beneficial to patients who have not experienced a heart attack. Anyone who has undergone a heart surgery or PCI will find cardiac rehab valuable for recovery and prevention of further problems. If you have a heart condition, particularly if you were recently discharged from the hospital, ask your health-care provider whether a cardiac rehabilitation program is right for you.

What Is a Stroke?

A stroke is sometimes called a "brain attack." It is similar to a heart attack in that the flow of blood and oxygen is interrupted to an area of the brain. When that happens, the area not receiving oxygenated blood is injured. Many strokes are caused by a blood clot in an artery in the brain; these types of strokes are called *embolic strokes*. Both embolisms and atherosclerosis may obstruct blood flow to the brain. Therefore, it's not surprising that many medications given to reduce clots in the heart are similar to those used in stroke management. Other types of strokes can occur if there is bleeding in the brain; these are called *hemorrhagic strokes*. The management of hemorrhagic strokes may be very different from that of heart attacks or embolic strokes because of the difference in the origin or cause.

As we have discussed, both strokes and heart disease are considered cardiovascular diseases. Together, they are the two biggest killers in our country. In fact, according to the Centers for Disease Control and Prevention, stroke is the third leading cause of death in the United States.

- Approximately 795, 000 Americans experience a stroke each year (601,000 new and 185,000 recurrent).
- Stroke accounts for 1 out of every 18 deaths in the United States (one every 40 seconds).
- From 1998 to 2008, the annual stroke death rate fell 34.8 percent

Warning Signs of a Stroke

As with heart attacks, it's very important to know the warning signs of a stroke and immediately seek emergency medical treatment. Strokes can cause permanent damage, including paralysis of certain extremities or an entire side of the body. They can also affect basic neurologic functions, such as thinking, understanding, and speaking. A severe stroke may also result in death. Unless a stroke is treated within hours of onset, there is little that can be done other than watching and waiting. Of course, just as with heart disease, prevention is your best defense against a stroke.

Some signs that a stroke is occurring include the following:
- sudden weakness (or numbness) of the face, arm, or leg, particularly on one side of the body
- sudden trouble with your vision
- sudden confusion; trouble speaking or understanding
- sudden onset of dizziness, difficulty walking, or loss of balance or coordination
- sudden severe headache

Stroke Treatment

Depending on the type of stroke, a neurologist, along with other health-care providers, will treat the stroke with careful monitoring and control of blood pressure. Testing usually includes imaging the brain with computerized tomography (CT) scans and/or magnetic resonance imaging (MRI). If an artery is blocked, clot-busting medications may be beneficial in restoring blood flow to the brain if it's identified early on. The same anticlotting medications used for some types of heart attacks may also be considered. For patients with hemorrhagic strokes, controlling blood pressure is important, in addition to stopping any ongoing bleeding. In some cases, surgery is required to stop the hemorrhage.

What Is a TIA?

A TIA is a transient ischemia attack, sometimes referred to as a mini-stroke. A TIA is like chest pain without having a heart attack; it's a warning sign that the brain is briefly not getting the oxygenated blood it needs. The symptoms are the same as stroke symptoms, but with the TIA the interruption of blood flow does not last long enough to cause permanent damage. Women who experience a TIA are at much higher risk for a stroke. Consequently, it does not matter if the symptoms are due to a TIA or a stroke: calling 911 and seeking immediate medical care is very important.

What Is Peripheral Arterial Disease?

When blood flow to the legs is blocked, the condition is called peripheral arterial disease (PAD). Just like your heart and brain, your extremities need oxygenated blood to work properly. As you might imagine, when the arteries in your legs are clogged, they begin to ache, and this discomfort will be become more severe as time goes on. If left untreated, circulation to the feet can be blocked entirely, and this may lead to amputation. Just as important, you are more likely to have a heart attack or stroke if you have PAD. So, it's vital that you seek treatment for this condition and make the necessary changes to prevent more serious events.

Warning signs and symptoms of PAD include:
- cramping, heaviness, fatigue, or aching of the buttocks, thighs, or calves when walking
- leg pain that occurs when you walk uphill, carry heavy loads, or increase your pace
- aching of the foot that worsens at night (when lying down) and feels better when you stand up or hang your foot off the bed
- leg pain that stops when you stand still or rest

We have covered a basic overview of many common heart problems. In the following chapters, we will go into more detail about some of these heart problems and then focus on how you can assess your risk for heart disease and take key prevention steps.

In addition to the heart, many other parts of our bodies may be negatively affected by atherosclerosis and lack of blood flow, including our intestines. So, you can see how important it is to keep your cardiovascular system in good health. Fortunately, the process of atherosclerosis and its effects can be prevented. Here's what you can do to get started:

- First and foremost, if you have experienced any of the warning signs or symptoms described here, talk to your health-care provider right away. Do not hesitate to ask for further testing or a second opinion if you feel it's necessary.
- Find out how women differ from men when it comes to heart disease (see chapter 4) so you can recognize and prevent problems.
- Learn about your risks for heart disease (see chapter 5) and how to manage those risks.

CHAPTER THREE

A Beautiful Rhythm

Dance to the rhythm of your heart and you will feel happiness like never before.

SIMRAN KHURANA

While coronary artery disease (CAD) accounts for the majority of heart attacks, problems with the heart's rhythm are also common, particularly among women. You can think of the heart's function—the process of blood entering the heart and being pumped out effectively—as a symphony, with your blood vessels, heart chambers, and valves all playing their parts in a precise rhythm. Like any symphony, this process needs a good conductor. The *conduction system* (also called the electrical system) serves that role; it's the electrical component of the heart that regulates your heartbeat. In other words, this system is your heart's natural pacemaker.

Through coordinated electrical impulses, the conduction system tells the heart what to do and establishes a rhythm. When this rhythm is disrupted, we experience arrhythmias or irregular heartbeats. Approximately one in three people will have some type of heart arrhythmia during their lifetime. These irregular heartbeats may feel like fluttering in your chest or neck, or cause the sensation of a skipped beat or pause. Some arrhythmias are so brief they don't change your heart rate, while others can cause your heart to beat too fast or too slow. Arrhythmias can cause a wide range of symptoms, from nothing at all to dizziness or light-headedness—and at the most extreme, heart attack or death.

While most arrhythmias are considered harmless and are left untreated, others can cause serious problems with the heart's function. When arrhythmias are severe or long-lasting, the heart may not be able to pump enough blood to the rest of the body, including the heart muscle itself, resulting in a heart attack. Although there are many types of arrhythmias, we will focus on the two most common conditions: atrial fibrillation and supraventricular arrhythmia.

Types of Arrhythmias

Bradycardia occurs when the heart beats **too slowly**—less than 60 beats per minute (60–100 beats per minute at rest is considered normal). For some people, a slow heart rate does not cause any problems. In fact, it can be a sign of being very fit. Athletes often have heart rates of less than 60 beats per minute. For other people, however, bradycardia signals a problem with the heart's electrical system. The heart's pacemaker may not be working correctly, or the electrical pathways may be disrupted. In severe cases, the heart beats so slowly that it does not pump enough blood to meet the body's needs, which can be life threatening.

Problematic bradycardia is more likely to occur during a person's advanced years and requires treatment. In addition to aging, a slow heart rate can be caused by:

- diseases that damage the heart's electrical system, including coronary artery disease, heart attacks, and certain infections
- conditions such as a low thyroid level or an electrolyte imbalance
- certain medications, such as those used for treating high blood pressure and arrhythmias

---

Symptoms of bradycardia include:

- dizziness or light-headedness
- shortness of breath (finding it harder to exercise)
- unusual fatigue
- chest pain or a feeling that your heart is pounding or fluttering (palpitations)
- confusion or trouble concentrating

Tachycardia is when the heart rate is **too fast**—more than 100 beats per minute. Certain types of tachycardia are normal—it may occur when we get excited or nervous, or drink too much caffeine, for instance. A rapid heartbeat can also be caused by:

- thyroid disease
- high fevers
- certain drugs, including asthma and allergy medications
- underlying heart disease, such as coronary artery disease and valve problems
- a heart attack

The main symptom of tachycardia is an awareness of a rapid heartbeat, or palpitations. Other symptoms may include:

- shortness of breath
- dizziness
- fainting
- chest pain
- severe anxiety

Atrial Fibrillation

Nearly three million Americans have experienced atrial fibrillation or "AFib," which is basically an abnormal heartbeat. Though it can affect anyone, this condition is much more common in the elderly. In fact, we expect the number of people with AFib to increase dramatically over the next several decades for two reasons. First, our population is aging, and we know that older folks are more likely to develop abnormal heartbeats. Second, the number of adults with hypertension is growing, and high blood pressure (especially if it's not well controlled) is a major risk factor for AFib. In addition to age and high blood pressure, other risk factors for developing atrial fibrillation include:

- heart disease, including valve problems and a history of heart attack and heart surgery
- chronic conditions such as thyroid problems and sleep apnea
- drinking alcohol, especially binge drinking (five or more drinks in two hours for men, and four drinks for women)
- Family history

Atrial fibrillation occurs when the top chambers of your heart, called the atria, do not beat regularly but rather "fibrillate," or quiver like gelatin, and do not coordinate with the bottom chambers (ventricles). This uncoordinated contraction is caused by impulses traveling down to the ventricles in an irregular way, making it difficult for blood to move to the ventricles effectively. An irregular pulse is one of the top signs that you are experiencing AFib. If the impulses that travel to the ventricles are too fast, you may also experience a rapid heart rate.

Symptoms of atrial fibrillation can include:

- palpitations or a rapid, irregular heart rate
- light-headedness or dizziness
- chest pain
- shortness of breath
- loss of consciousness or fainting

If you experience any of these symptoms, you must seek medical attention right away. Chances are, your heart is beating too rapidly and you need medications to help slow the rate down. When your heart beats too fast, you may not get enough blood into your coronary arteries, which means the heart muscle does not receive enough oxygen. As you now know, this lack of oxygen can lead to a heart attack.

AFib and Stroke

Many people who experience AFib are also at an increased risk for stroke. Since blood is not flowing properly through the atria during AFib, there is a chance that blood will pool and form a clot. If a piece of the clot breaks off and travels to the brain, that can lead to a stroke. Therefore, in addition to prescribing medications to slow your heart rate down, your physician may also assess your risk for stroke.

If you develop AFib, you are considered high-risk for stroke if you have a history of hypertension, diabetes, heart failure, or past stroke, or are over 65 years of age. Being a woman and/or having a history of heart disease or other vascular disease are also considered risk factors for stroke with AFib. With each additional risk factor, your chance of stroke multiplies. So, it's not uncommon for patients with AFib who also have several risk factors to be put on a blood thinner, such as warfarin or Coumadin. Taking a blood thinner can lower your risk for stroke by about 60 percent when you have AFib. For younger patients, and those with no risk factors, aspirin may be a better alternative. Women with periodic or paroxysmal atrial fibrillation are at the same risk for stroke as someone who has chronic AFib, and therefore may require a blood thinner, in addition to other treatments.

Recently, newer medications have been approved by the FDA to reduce stroke risk in patients who have AFib. The benefit of these drugs, which include dabigatran, rivaroxaban, and apixaban, is less frequent blood checks, which are required regularly when taking traditional blood thinners. While these drugs are still new, results look promising and give patients with AFib more options. The bottom line: If you have AFib, it's important to discuss your risk for stroke and medication alternatives with your physician.

Chronic vs. Periodic AFib

Atrial fibrillation can be tricky. Some people experience AFib followed by a return to normal sinus rhythm. When the irregular heartbeat doesn't last and the heart returns to a normal rhythm, we call this *paroxysmal atrial fibrillation*. It's not uncommon for people with paroxysmal atrial fibrillation to go back and forth from normal to irregular heartbeats, in and out of AFib. In this case, your physician will typically prescribe medications that help maintain a normal heart rhythm. These are called antiarrhythmic medications. There are several types of antiarrhythmic drugs—each one uses a different method for keeping your heartbeat within a normal range, and each one comes with unique side effects. It may take some time, working with your physician, to find a medication that works well for you with minimal side effects. Often, a heart rhythm specialist, called an electrophysiologist, is consulted to help with such arrhythmias. Electrophysiologists are cardiologists who have received advanced training in heart rhythms.

An alternative to medication is a procedure called *ablation*. Ablations are performed generally by electrophysiologists but sometimes by surgeons. The type of arrhythmia and the presence of other heart disease determine what type of procedure is recommended. A catheter is inserted into a specific area of the heart. Then, energy is directed through the catheter to areas of the heart muscle that cause the abnormal heartbeat. This energy disconnects the source of the arrhythmia from the rest of the heart. It can also be used to disconnect the electrical pathway between the upper chambers (atria) and the lower chambers (ventricles). Ablation procedures may be minimally invasive or may involve traditional open heart surgery, and may be combined with other procedures such as bypass surgery, valve repair, or valve replacement. Before undergoing any procedure to correct an arrhythmia, it's important to discuss both the pros and cons, including possible complications.

Supraventricular Arrhythmia

Technically, any rapid, irregular heartbeat that originates above the ventricles is a supraventricular tachycardia (SVT), including atrial fibrillation. While AFib is the most common type, there are many others. Sometimes the heart impulse starts in the atria, but not from the area of the heart that normally begins the beat. In other cases, the impulse starts out normally, but is disrupted along the pathway. Consequently, the impulses travel too fast and create a circle of rapid beats, which resembles a continuous loop of electrical current. The rapid heartbeat that results from this loop can be very uncomfortable. Fortunately, the majority of SVTs can be managed with medications, or procedures that "disconnect" the abnormal impulse or pathway.

Many things can trigger an SVT, including thyroid problems, excessive alcohol, smoking, illegal drugs such as cocaine, lung disease such as COPD, sleep apnea, and emotional stressors. In a large number of cases, lifestyle changes can eliminate or control these types of arrhythmias. Though SVTs are not generally life threatening, they may cause worsening heart function if sustained for long periods of time.

Pregnancy can also increase SVT episodes in some women. If this occurs, medication can be used to control the arrhythmias during the pregnancy, without danger to mother or child. However, it's important to let your physician know if you have a history of SVT prior to becoming pregnant so the condition can be monitored effectively.

Keeping Pace

Each of us has a natural pacemaker in our heart's conduction system, which regulates our heartbeat. As we've seen, when this system is disrupted, our heartbeats can be abnormal. When the disruption in the electrical system becomes permanent or severe (due to age or heart disease), a cardiac pacemaker may be necessary. This small, sophisticated electronic device is implanted under the skin to help regulate the heartbeat. Pacemakers don't take over the work of the heart; they merely help regulate the timing and sequence of your heartbeat.

Pacemakers are useful in many cardiac conditions, but are most commonly employed in patients who have very slow heart rates (bradycardia). The device monitors the heart's activity, and if the heart rate becomes too slow, it transmits a tiny electrical signal to the heart muscle, causing it to contract. It can also coordinate beats between the upper and lower chambers of the heart. By keeping an appropriate heart rate, a pacemaker can help alleviate the symptoms of a slow heart rate, including weakness, fatigue, light-headedness, dizziness, and loss of consciousness. And, because pacemakers are "programmable," your physician can change the rate at which yours paces your heart to achieve optimal results.

Take a Step

For the most part, our hearts perform their function without notice—beating in a beautiful, life-sustaining rhythm to which we grow accustomed. So, it can be very disconcerting to feel a change in that rhythm. Though most arrhythmias are harmless, you should never assume that nothing is wrong. Any change in your heartbeat warrants a visit to your health-care provider to rule out any serious problems. Even if your arrhythmia is deemed "innocent," medications can keep your heart in sync and make you feel more comfortable.

- If you are experiencing, or have experienced, any of the symptoms we've discussed, including a rapid, racing heartbeat, dizziness, shortness of breath, fainting or chest pain, seek medical attention right away. A simple EKG can often diagnose the problem. In some cases, you will be asked to wear a Holter monitor, which is a machine that continuously records the heart's rhythms. The monitor is usually worn for 24 to 48 hours during normal activity, while electrodes attached to your chest record your heart's electrical activity and identify any abnormal rhythms.

- If you're a woman with a history of high blood pressure and are experiencing abnormal heart rhythms, talk to your physician about your increased risk for stroke. Taking blood thinners can decrease your stroke risk significantly.

- Avoid energy drinks, diet pills, and other products containing excessive caffeine and other chemical stimulants. These products may cause tachycardia (rapid heart rate) and, in extreme cases, put you at risk for a heart attack.

CHAPTER FOUR

Not for Men Only

With man the world is his heart, with woman the heart is her world.

BETTY GRABLE

If you ask a woman what disease she fears most, chances are her answer will be "breast cancer." While breast cancer affects many women, heart disease is actually the leading cause of death among women of all ages—taking the lives of six times as many women as breast cancer each year. In fact, heart attacks kill 267,000 American women annually, more than all forms of cancer combined. Further sobering is the fact that every year since 1984, heart attacks have killed more women in the United States than men.

Those statistics debunk the long-standing belief that heart disease is primarily a male health issue. For the first 80 years or so of the twentieth century, medical experts believed that estrogen provided women with lasting protection against heart disease and, consequently, focused their research on men. Estrogen does afford premenopausal women with a certain amount of defense, but by the age of 65, women "catch up" with men regarding cardiovascular problems. Furthermore, estrogen is not a magic shield—many women under the age of 65 develop heart disease. Of the approximately 435,000 American women who have heart attacks each year, 83,000 are under the age of 65, and 35,000 are under the age of 55. Women who experience heart attacks under the age of 50 are twice as likely as men to have fatal events.

Why is heart disease such a serious and growing threat among women? Unfortunately, there is still a sizable gap in knowledge. Though both research and awareness have increased, we still have a long way to go to educate women and health-care professionals. Surveys show that awareness of heart attack warning signs is still low among women, especially minority women. In a 2009 study, only half of the women participating correctly identified pain in the neck, shoulders, or arms as potential symptoms of a heart attack. This may explain why only 50 percent of women actually experiencing a heart attack call 911! More importantly, some reports suggest that women's heart attack symptoms are ignored or misdiagnosed by many emergency and medical professionals.

Women are also less likely to discuss heart disease with their physicians. If I could encourage women to do just one thing, it would be this: **include a discussion of your cardiac risk factors at every physical exam!** And if you are experiencing or have experienced any early warning signs (see "Warning Signs ...," page 54), seek medical attention immediately. Do not assume you're too young, too healthy, or the wrong gender to have heart problems. If you experience warning signs, always ask "could it be my heart?"—even if you receive another diagnosis such as anxiety, heartburn, or muscle strain.

We may soon see an increase in heart disease among women (and men) mainly due to unhealthy lifestyle choices. As our population becomes more sedentary and obese, and as we continue to consume diets high in saturated fats, sugar, and salt, we dramatically increase our risk for heart disease and stroke. Furthermore, with the general aging of our population, we will have more Americans living with heart disease than ever before. And, when women begin to suffer from diabetes, high cholesterol, and high blood pressure earlier in life, they significantly increase their chances of

Warning Signs Women Should Never Ignore

Women are more likely to experience early warning signs before a heart attack. In fact, about 80 percent of women report early warning signs, versus 50 percent of men. Women's heart attack symptoms may also be more subtle than those experienced by men. Recognizing these symptoms and seeking immediate medical attention can save your life! When a heart attack strikes, getting medical help within the first hour reduces the risk of dying by 50 percent. If you have any of these warning signs, call 911.

- **Chest pain**—The majority of women having a heart attack do experience chest pain. It may not be the crushing, explosive pain that many men report, but any sudden, severe, or persisting chest pain warrants concern.
- **Unusual fatigue**—In one study of female heart attack survivors, about 70 percent reported extreme fatigue in the days and weeks prior to the attack. They felt too tired to complete simple tasks, such as making the bed or walking to the mailbox.
- **Shortness of breath**—Many women report gasping as if they'd just run a long distance or having difficulty talking during a heart attack. In some cases, this shortness of breath can occur days or even weeks prior to a cardiac event.
- **Nausea or dizziness**—Women frequently feel nauseous, vomit, or feel like they might faint during a heart attack. The symptoms may also feel like heartburn or an upset stomach.
- **Profuse sweating**—A heart attack may cause a woman to be suddenly drenched in sweat for no reason. Oftentimes, women feel both hot and cold (clammy) during an attack.
- **Non-chest pain**—Instead of a crushing pain in the chest, many women develop less severe pain in the upper back, shoulders, neck, jaw, or arm.
- **Anxiety**—You can call it "women's intuition"—many women experience a feeling of "impending doom" or intense fear before or during a heart attack.

developing heart disease earlier in life. So, although women and men do not always experience heart attacks the same way, there are more similarities than differences between us when it comes to heart disease. For instance, the best course of treatment is the same for both sexes: prevention!

However, since there are some differences in the types of heart problems women encounter and the way our bodies respond, it's important to understand those variances. In this chapter, we will look at a few of the heart conditions that are more common in women than men, as well as how hormones affect our hearts.

Women Under the Microscope

Our knowledge of heart disease in women has significantly improved in recent years due to the inclusion of women in more clinical trials, along with major landmark studies of female populations. These studies have improved our understanding of the similarities of cardiovascular disease among women and men, as well as the potential differences. For example, the Nurses' Health Study, a long-term project that followed over 100,000 women, gathered data on many factors that influence women's health. The results of this study have provided important findings related to heart disease in women. In fact, we have referenced the Nurses' Health Study throughout the book.

Another important clinical trial was the Women's Health Study, which examined the use of aspirin for primary prevention of heart disease in women. Because aspirin therapy has proven effective in men, it was assumed that aspirin also worked for women. However, this trial showed that aspirin did not lower the risk for heart attacks in women, particularly younger women. Today, the current guidelines for women do not recommend aspirin for primary

> While men tend to accumulate plaque in one or two areas of the coronary arteries, women are more likely to build plaque throughout the arterial system. Women usually have plaque in smaller coronary arteries, as well.

prevention of heart disease in females under the age of 65 years.

The Women's Ischemia Syndrome Evaluation (WISE), which studied women who were referred for coronary angiography (a procedure that uses special dye and X-rays to see how blood flows through the arteries in the heart), also showed some important gender differences. For instance, the WISE investigators found that many women have nonobstructive coronary artery disease (CAD) as opposed to major blockages in the arteries. Despite having no significant blockages, the women in the WISE study who reported chest pain were at a higher risk for heart attacks compared to women who did not report chest pain.

Thanks to this and other studies, we have improved our understanding of diagnostic testing in women. As a result, we now know that women are more likely to develop several conditions that affect the heart, including microvascular disease, coronary vasospasm, and broken heart syndrome.

Microvascular Disease

Coronary microvascular disease, also known as small vessel disease or Syndrome X, occurs when the small arteries in the heart become narrow and inflexible. Normally, these blood vessels expand during activity, allowing more oxygen into your blood. When these small vessels cannot expand, blood flow to the heart muscle may be reduced, resulting in chest pain. Women with microvascular disease are also more likely to have a condition called *endothelial dysfunction*. The endothelium is a smooth, tile-like layer of specialized cells that line the inner walls of your blood vessels. This lining performs many important functions, including keeping blood in and toxins out, as well as helping the arteries remain flexible.

Microvascular disease is more prevalent in women and people with diabetes, although the reason for this is still unclear. Though sometimes difficult to detect, the condition is treatable. The most common symptom of microvascular disease is chest pain or pressure, which may be more noticeable when you are walking or climbing stairs. Stress may also trigger chest discomfort. While these symptoms are similar to angina, which is caused by blockages in the coronary arteries, patients with this condition do not have significant blockages in larger arteries. In fact, though women with microvascular disease may have an abnormal stress test, significant blockages in the three major arteries are not detected when a coronary angiogram is performed. So why are these women having chest pain?

It is not completely clear why some patients have symptoms due to microvascular disease. In women, there is some evidence to suggest that estrogen levels may play a role in this syndrome since most of these patients are perimenopausal or postmenopausal. Some scientists also think the tissues that line the chambers of the heart may be receiving less blood flow. It's possible this reduced blood flow is due to damage in the lining of the blood vessels (i.e., endothelial dysfunction). As we know, many cardiac risk factors can harm the lining of blood vessels over time.

Although there is currently no specific recommended testing for microvascular disease, studies suggest that a cardiac MRI, which looks at blood flow to the heart, including the small vessels, can help detect the condition. Once the problem is diagnosed, the overall prognosis is very good. Women with microvascular disease have a lower risk for heart attacks compared to women (or men) with significant blockages in their coronary arteries. Still, chest pain is cause for concern and increases one's risk for heart disease compared to those with no symptoms. Therefore, reducing symptoms with medication along with lifestyle modifications is the main course of treatment.

When deciding on treatment, it's important to work closely with your physician, as medications can have varying results. What works well for some women may not work well for others. For example, nitroglycerin may reduce chest pain in some women with microvascular disease, but not for others. Beta-blockers, ACE inhibitors, and even certain types of anti-depressants have all been used to treat this type of chest pain. In other words, it may take some trial and error to find the best solution.

In addition to medication, women with microvascular disease should aggressively modify cardiac risk factors. They need to be careful, for example, about controlling blood pressure and reducing cholesterol. A healthy diet, regular exercise, smoking cessation, and stress reduction may all assist in reducing chest pain and improve your overall risk for developing heart disease. If you suspect you have microvascular disease, talking with your physician is the first step in evaluation.

Coronary Vasospasm

Coronary vasospasm, also termed coronary vasospastic angina or Prinzmetal's angina, occurs when the coronary artery goes into spasm—a sudden, involuntary contraction that causes constriction of the artery. Patients with this condition have chest discomfort that has been described as crushing pain that may radiate to the arm, neck, or jaw. It can affect young and old, male or female, though it seems to occur more commonly in women. Coronary vasospasm is often thought to happen more frequently at night or at rest; however, some patients report chest discomfort with exercise or other activity. Again, stress can also trigger a spasm.

Although coronary vasospasm causes symptoms that are very similar to angina, testing shows little to no atherosclerosis or blockage. Studies suggest that the smooth muscle in the coronary artery is hyperactive. Once again, the problem stems from the cells lining the walls of the arteries. For some reason, these endothelial cells do not respond correctly to natural chemicals secreted by the body to expand the arteries; instead of expanding, they actually contract or constrict. Substances such as acetylcholine, serotonin, histamine, and noradrenaline (all neurotransmitters) can provoke a spasm, which leads us to believe that an imbalance in the nervous system may play a role in this condition.

In addition, coronary vasospasm may be associated with other disorders, including microvascular disease, Raynaud's syndrome (a condition that causes extremities such as your fingers and toes to feel numb and be discolored in response to cold temperatures or stress), and migraine headaches. At their root, all of these conditions involve limited blood circulation in the smaller arteries and, interestingly, affect more women than men. Perhaps this is because women have naturally smaller arteries than men.

This condition can be difficult to diagnose. Both EKGs and stress tests may be normal during an episode. Administering nitroglycerin can often relax the artery and relieve the symptoms instantly, whereas symptoms caused by a clot would not be resolved completely. To confirm a diagnosis, a coronary angiogram is necessary. Once diagnosed, symptoms are treated with medication, including statin therapy, calcium channel blockers, and nitrates. Reviewing other medications with your physician is important since some experts suggest that certain drugs such as beta-blockers (propranolol) and some migraine therapies (sumatriptan) can actually trigger coronary vasospasm.

Cigarette smoking is also considered a trigger for coronary vasospasm and should be stopped immediately if this condition is suspected.

In general, most patients with coronary vasospasm do not have heart attacks, but there is a risk for myocardial damage if the spasm is severe and reduced blood flow to an area of the heart is prolonged. This could result in a heart attack if not treated.

Broken Heart Syndrome

Also known as stress-induced cardiomyopathy and takotsubo cardiomyopathy, broken heart syndrome is another condition that occurs more often in women than men. The syndrome gets its name from a distinctively shaped Japanese octopus trap called a takotsubo. When this syndrome happens, the heart swells and looks similar to one of these traps. The term "broken heart syndrome" is derived from its cause: It's believed that extreme psychological stress, such as the sudden loss of a loved one, causes a massive surge in stress hormones such as adrenaline. It may be that stress along with increases in hormones produced by the adrenal glands weakens the heart muscle. We sometimes see a similar phenomenon in the intensive care unit (ICU) when patients are very sick with noncardiac illnesses; the heart muscle can weaken for a short time.

The truth is that no one is really sure why broken heart syndrome occurs. It's also unclear why certain areas of the heart, such as the left ventricular walls, are affected more than other areas. The fact that women are more vulnerable to this condition is also a mystery. Most of the women who experience broken heart syndrome are postmenopausal, which suggests that changes in estrogen or other sex hormones may be a contributing factor. However, no detailed studies have been conducted to verify this theory.

Broken heart syndrome can be very frightening since it mimics a heart attack, complete with chest pain or discomfort and labored breathing. Even an EKG suggests that the patient is having a heart attack. Yet, when a coronary angiogram (catheterization) is performed, the arteries appear normal. In severe cases, this syndrome can cause heart failure. Fortunately, it is usually resolved over time—with complete recovery in several weeks.

To alleviate the discomfort, medications are typically prescribed to help the left ventricle pump effectively (if function is impaired), just as with other forms of heart failure. Many cardiologists also use beta-blockers to protect against future episodes, particularly until the heart muscle gets stronger. However, until more research is conducted, the best way to manage the condition long-term is still unclear.

Sudden Cardiac Death

Though the term is terrifying to both sexes, sudden cardiac death has different implications for men and women. In general, women have lower rates of this fatal event compared to men—even among women who are considered at high risk for heart disease. However, women who experience sudden cardiac death are more likely to have no prior history of heart problems, which means that sudden cardiac death may be the first and only sign of a heart attack for women.

Most often, it is caused by a severe arrhythmia, such as ventricular tachycardia or ventricular fibrillation, which occurs when the heart muscle is not getting enough oxygen. Once robbed of sufficient oxygen, the heart simply stops beating. Since there is no way to predict this type of event, knowing your cardiovascular risk factors, such as blood pressure and cholesterol as well as modifying these risks, is the best defense.

Hormones and Your Heart

What do we really know about estrogen? Estrogen, along with testosterone and progesterone, is a chemical substance or hormone produced primarily by our ovaries (it's also produced by the body's fat tissue). Estrogen, testosterone, and progesterone are considered sex hormones because they are involved in the growth, maintenance, and repair of our reproductive tissues. The level of these hormones in our body can vary from day to day, hour to hour, and even minute to minute. Of course, more significant changes in hormone levels occur during a woman's menstrual cycle.

As a woman ages, levels of sex hormones, particularly estrogen and progesterone, decline. Once the ovaries stop producing eggs and a woman transitions through menopause, estrogen levels drop dramatically. Though natural, this process is very complex, and although our current understanding has improved immeasurably, there is still a great deal about this transition that is unknown. We do know, however, that postmenopausal women are more likely to develop heart disease.

It's long been observed that women tend to experience heart events about ten years later than men. The hypothesis for the explanation of this age difference has been that estrogen protects the heart until it declines during menopause. Estrogen appears to lower LDL (bad) cholesterol levels, which lessens your chance of developing atherosclerosis and, therefore, heart disease. In addition, large studies observed that women who were taking hormone replacement therapy (HRT) after menopause had a lower risk for heart disease compared to women who were not on HRT. The data suggested that HRT was "cardio protective." But this was an incorrect assumption.

Since women who take hormones may or may not have additional risk factors that differ from those of women who don't take HRT, it was impossible to confirm the benefits of taking estrogen without a more controlled study. The Heart and Estrogen/Progestin Replacement Study (HERS) looked specifically at hormone replacement therapy among women with a prior history of heart disease and found some surprising results. For women who had recently had a heart attack, HRT actually increased the risk for future cardiac events.

This led to other large investigations such as the Women's Health Initiative (WHI), which examined the effect of HRT on women with no prior history of heart disease. This study divided women into two groups: one taking estrogen and progesterone if they still had a uterus and ovaries, and the second taking only estrogen if they had had a hysterectomy. When the group taking both estrogen and progesterone (or placebo) was found to have an increased risk for stroke, coronary heart disease, and blood clots, in addition to a higher incidence of breast cancer, the study was halted. (The study did note a reduced risk for bone fractures and colon cancer.) In the group taking estrogen alone (or placebo), there was an increased risk for stroke, while no increase or decrease in heart disease was observed.

What does all this mean? As a result of these larger and more recent studies, HRT is *not* recommended for prevention of cardiovascular disease. Furthermore, hormone therapy is discouraged for women who have a history of cardiovascular disease.

It's important to note that most of these studies used only one type of estrogen and progesterone. Some scientists and clinicians believe that other types of estrogen may not present the same risk for cardiovascular disease. In addition, these studies enrolled women who were postmenopausal, which means they were older than many women who are considering HRT. When investigators looked at results by age, it appears that younger women (less than 60 years old) do not have the same risk for cardiovascular disease when taking HRT as older women do, which leads some to believe that the benefits of estrogen (i.e., lowering LDL cholesterol and improving endothelial function) may be greater among younger women. Since estrogen can also increase triglyceride levels, blood clots, and inflammation, it could be that these factors are more detrimental to older women.

By now, you've probably surmised that there are many unan-swered questions regarding HRT and heart disease! This has led to many confusing messages regarding HRT in the media and, in some cases, among health-care professionals. Since the risks and benefits related to hormone therapy are different for every woman, there is no definitive answer. My advice to women who are con-sidering HRT is to have a thorough discussion with your physician about specific risks for cardiovascular disease in relation to your particular health situation. If you are considering HRT to reduce your risk of bone fractures, ask your physician about alternative therapies. If you are thinking about taking hormones to ease menopausal symptoms such as hot flashes, be sure to ask about the duration of the therapy. Most health-care professionals recom-mend short-term (under five years) use if HRT is prescribed. Un-fortunately, many women find that hot flashes and night sweats return once HRT is stopped.

The bottom line: The best protection against heart disease, both before and after menopause, is reducing and/or controlling cardiac risk factors and adopting a healthy lifestyle.

Take a Step

Heart disease is an equal-opportunity health problem. As a woman, you should be aware of both the similarities and differences of heart disease symptoms between the sexes and never hesitate to seek medical attention if you experience these warning signs. Protect your heart and your life by:
- Discussing cardiac risk factors with your physician at every exam.
- Knowing your numbers—blood pressure, cholesterol levels, and blood glucose—and keeping them in a healthy range.
- Asking "could it be my heart?" if you experience cardiac symptoms, even if you receive a different diagnosis.
- Calling 911 if you experience any heart attack warning signs.

CHAPTER FIVE

Assessing Your Risk

*Never let the odds keep you from doing what you know in
your heart you were meant to do.*

H. JACKSON BROWN JR.

There are no crystal balls when it comes to heart
health. Even with today's advanced science, we cannot predict,
with complete accuracy, whether or when someone will develop
cardiovascular disease. However, we have become very knowledge-
able about the factors that significantly increase or decrease our
risks. Since prevention is the most powerful weapon against heart
disease, understanding what these risk factors are and how to manage them is your first line of defense. The leading risk factors for
heart disease are:

- age and gender
- family history
- hypertension or high blood pressure
- cholesterol levels (high LDL cholesterol and low HDL
  cholesterol)
- diabetes
- smoking

- excess weight
- sedentary lifestyle

   While certain factors such as gender, age, and family history are beyond our control, there is still much we can do to improve our odds. It's true that having one risk factor, such as age, may be enough to cause a heart attack or stroke, but far more often, it's a combination of influences that lead to heart problems—particularly *premature* heart disease. As you might expect, the more of these risk factors you possess, the greater your chances of developing heart disease. For instance, being inactive and overweight as well as a smoker puts you at a much higher risk than someone who is struggling with weight alone. The following chapters focus on each of the major risk factors that can be managed, including high blood pressure, cholesterol, diabetes, diet, exercise, and stress. What about the risk factors you can't change?

Family History

A patient once told me she felt "destined to have heart problems," due to her strong family history. Since she was also wrestling with some lifestyle issues, it seemed to me she had given up before the fight began. You can't change your genes, but genes are not destiny—they are only part of the equation. My advice to this patient was to consider her family history a challenge and change what she could. If you have a family history of heart disease, it's even more important for you to manage the risk factors you can control.

   Physicians define a "family history of premature heart disease" as having a first-degree female relative (mother, sister, or daughter) under the age of 65 or a first-degree male relative (father, brother, or son) under the age of 55 who has heart disease. If your parents have heart disease, you are more likely to develop it—but it's not guaranteed. Again, there is much you can do to lessen your risk, including having annual checkups.

Age and Gender

We've already discussed the fact that heart disease is the leading cause of death for women and is no longer considered a male-only health issue. However, men are at greater risk of developing heart disease at an earlier age. From the age of 45, a man's risk for heart problems begins to increase and continues to escalate with age. Unfortunately, statistics show that by the age of 65, half of all American men are likely to suffer from heart disease.

As we've seen, women appear to benefit from some protection provided by estrogen before menopause. After menopause, this defense disappears, which means women who are 55 and older are at an increased risk for heart disease. This risk also intensifies with age. By the age of 65, a third of all American women are likely to develop heart disease. Clearly, women with more risk factors increase the threat. In the next section, we will discuss how clinicians can calculate your risk of developing heart disease and stroke based on your health and lifestyle.

What Is Your Risk for Heart Disease?

Most physicians use specific risk prediction tools to assess a patient's probability of developing heart disease (the next best thing to a crystal ball). We use these tools to determine how aggressive to be when treating risk factors such as elevated cholesterol levels. For example, if a woman has diabetes and is currently smoking, her risk for heart disease over the next ten years is much higher than that of a woman of similar age who does not have diabetes and is a nonsmoker. In this scenario, the woman who is at high risk will have a lower target for LDL (bad) cholesterol than the woman with less risk. In other words, these risk prediction tools help us establish treatment guidelines.

In the United States, current guidelines include the use of the Framingham Risk Score. This is the tool many health-care providers use to evaluate a woman's overall heart disease risk. In addition, data from Harvard's Women's Health Study were used to develop another prediction tool called the Reynolds Risk Score. Together, these are the most commonly used risk assessment tools in the United States.

You can find both tools online and calculate your personal risk for heart disease, either on your own or with the assistance of your health-care provider. Keep in mind that these tools are for women who have no prior history of heart disease. If you have heart disease, your risk for future events is elevated, and you should therefore be working aggressively with your physician to manage all risk factors, such as lowering blood pressure and keeping cholesterol in check.

The Framingham Risk Score

This tool is based on data from the Framingham Heart Study, which collected detailed information on the population of a town in Massachusetts over many decades. By following the health of these men and women over the years, the investigators were able to identify specific risk factors that were highly predictive of the development of heart disease. The Framingham Risk Score is used to estimate your heart disease risk over the next ten years and provides unique scores for men and women. It has proven so effective that guidelines written by experts from the American Heart Association and the American College of Cardiology are based on its results.

The Framingham Risk Score calculator is easy to use (see the web link at the end of this section). You simply supply information regarding your age, LDL and HDL cholesterol levels, and blood pressure, along with your diabetes and smoking status. If you use the calculator, you'll notice that age is the strongest predictor of heart disease—but the other factors are more important to understand, because they are the ones you can change! For example, if you're a smoker, try calculating your risk for heart disease using your correct smoking status and then recalculate your risk as a nonsmoker. The difference in scores gives you the approximate risk reduction you achieve by not smoking.

In general, a woman who has a 10 percent or lower risk for heart disease as calculated by the Framingham Risk Score is considered low risk. A woman who has a risk score between 10 and 20 percent is thought to be at an intermediate risk for heart events. And, a woman who has a score of 20 percent or greater is considered high risk.

In addition to this risk calculator, the Framingham investigators developed several other prediction tools. Since stroke is so prevalent among U.S. adults, a second model was created to predict all cardiovascular events, including stroke. The General Cardiovascular Disease Risk Score uses the same factors as the original Framingham Risk Score, but also includes body mass index (BMI), which takes weight into account.

The investigators also understood that our long-term or lifetime risk for heart attack and stroke is very important. Ten years, particularly when someone is young, does not allow for prediction of cardiac events when we are elderly. Therefore, they developed the Framingham Cardiovascular 30-Year Risk Tool that, as the name implies, assesses your risk over a 30-year span. This tool is particularly helpful for women who do not develop cardiovascular problems until later in life. By monitoring their risk factors from a younger age, it allows them to intervene earlier to lower blood pressure or cholesterol levels, thus preventing future events.

To learn more about these tools, you can visit the Framingham Study web site. There are several risk calculators, including the original 10-year risk score, the risk score for both heart disease and stroke, and a 30-year risk score:

- The Framingham Risk Score
  www.framinghamheartstudy.org/risk/coronary.html
- The General Cardiovascular Disease Risk Score
  www.framinghamheartstudy.org/risk/gencardio.html
- The Cardiovascular Disease Risk Score – 30-year risk
  www.framinghamheartstudy.org/risk/cardiovascular30.html

To calculate your personal risk score, go to the online Framingham calculator: http://hp2010.nhlbihin.net/atpiii/calculator.asp or visit the National Institutes of Health site, which includes the Framingham 10-year risk calculator.

The Reynolds Risk Score

The Reynolds Risk Score is similar to the Framingham Risk Score, with the exception of two factors: family history and C-reactive protein (a marker of inflammation determined by a blood test). After finding that individuals with high normal levels of C-reactive protein (CRP) were at increased risk for heart events, investigators developed the Reynolds Risk Score to incorporate CRP. This makes sense, since we know that inflammation can affect atherosclerotic plaque and therefore increase a woman's risk for a heart attack. The addition of CRP may help identify some adults at high risk who are not recognized by the traditional Framingham Risk Score.

While current guidelines do not suggest the routine measurement of CRP, it may be recommended for individuals who have several other risk factors.

In addition to heart disease, the Reynolds Risk Score also helps to predict the possibility of stroke. While both tools predict events over a ten-year period, the Reynolds tool groups women by risk level, with low being a less than 5 percent chance of cardiac events (over ten years). Low to moderate is defined as a risk between 5 and 10 percent, and moderate to high risk is specified as 10 to 20 percent. A score of 20 percent or more indicates a high risk for cardiovascular disease.

The web site for the Reynolds Risk Score is www.reynolds riskscore.org

Take a Step

Tools such as the Framingham and Reynolds risk scores not only predict who is most likely to develop cardiovascular disease, but also indicate who is most likely to benefit from prevention—and that's the key. Knowing your personal risk factors and learning how to reduce or manage them can lessen your chances of developing heart disease considerably. Here's what you can do:

- Assessing your risk begins with a visit to your health-care provider to obtain important information regarding your cholesterol levels, blood pressure, and, in some cases, blood glucose levels and BMI.
- Armed with these numbers, you can calculate your risk for developing cardiovascular disease using the Framingham or Reynolds risk score calculators. If your risk is slightly elevated to moderate, now is the time to make some changes. In the following chapters, you will learn how to lower blood pressure, improve your cholesterol profile, control blood sugar, follow a heart-healthy diet, increase your activity level, and manage stress. If your risk is moderate to high, it's time to talk to your physician about using medications to help reduce the threat to your heart, in conjunction with lifestyle changes.

Framingham Risk Score for Women

Age	Points	Age	Points
20–34	-7	55–59	8
35–39	-3	60–64	10
40–44	0	65–69	12
45–49	3	70–74	14
50–54	6	75–79	16

HDL	Points	HDL	Points
≥60	-1	40–49	1
50–59	0	<40	2

Total Cholesterol	Points at Ages 20–39	Points at Ages 40–49	Points at Ages 50–59	Points at Ages 60–69	Points at Ages 70–79
<160	0	0	0	0	0
160–199	4	3	2	1	1
200–239	8	6	4	2	1
240–279	11	8	5	3	2
≥280	13	10	7	4	2
Nonsmoker	0	0	0	0	0
Smoker	9	7	4	2	1

Systolic BP	If Untreated	If Treated
<120	0	0
120–129	1	3
130–139	2	4
140–159	3	5
≥160	4	6

Point Total	10-Year Risk	Point Total	10-Year Risk
<9	<1%	17	5%
9	1%	18	6%
10	1%	19	8%
11	1%	20	11%
12	1%	21	14%
13	2%	22	17%
14	2%	23	22%
15	3%	24	27%
16	4%	≥25	≥30%

JANE'S STORY

Jane is a 55-year-old woman who smokes about a half a pack of cigarettes a day and suffers from high blood pressure. Though her doctor has told her repeatedly that she is at an increased risk for heart disease, she never really understood what that meant. However, as a retired math teacher, Jane understands numbers well. So, when she attended a community lecture on women's health issues and heard about the Framingham Risk Score she was intrigued. After a quick search on the Internet, she found the Framingham Risk Score calculator on the National Institutes of Health web site. Since she had recently had her cholesterol and blood pressure checked, she was able to enter the following numbers into the calculator:

- Her age of 55 years gave her 8 points.
- Her smoking status gave her 4 points.
- Her recent blood pressure level was 145 (systolic), while currently on medication for her hypertension. This gave her 5 points.
- Jane is overweight and does not exercise. Consequently her HDL is low (<40 mg/dL). This gives her 2 points.
- In addition, her total cholesterol is >200 mg/dL, which gives her 4 points.

Total points = 23

A point total of 23 puts Jane's risk for a cardiovascular event in the next 10 years at 22 percent. Since a risk of 20 or more is considered high, this was an eye-opening moment for Jane. She realized that her doctor's concerns were valid and that she needed to make some changes to reduce her risk.

As Jane reviewed the risk factors, she noticed that she received the most points for her age. Since she couldn't change that, she focused on the modifiable factors. Being a smoker added four points (as well as a greater chance of developing other serious health issues), so that's where she began her efforts. It wasn't easy, but Jane was able to quit smoking with the support of her family. Not only did she feel better, but when she recalculated her risk score, she found that her risk for cardiovascular events had dropped to 8 percent over the next ten years. Encouraged, she decided to tackle another health problem.

By better controlling her blood pressure through diet and exercise, along with her medications, Jane realized she could further reduce her risk. In addition, Jane's physician told her that with exercise and weight loss, she could not only lower her blood pressure but also increase her HDL (good) cholesterol (see chapter 7). After several months of following a heart-healthy diet and walking for 20 to 30 minutes each day, Jane was happy to find that both her hypertension and cholesterol profile had improved. Armed with these new numbers, Jane recalculated her risk score and found that she had dropped into the low-risk category. Now, those were numbers she could live with!

CHAPTER SIX

Under Pressure

Sometimes the heart sees what is invisible to the eye.

H. JACKSON BROWN JR.

When was the last time you had your blood pressure checked? Most of us only have our blood pressure taken when we visit the doctor's office, which may not be regularly. If you've skipped annual physicals and haven't been ill enough to see a doctor, you could have had high blood pressure (also known as hypertension) for years without knowing it. Hypertension can sneak up on you. In fact, it's sometimes called the "silent killer," because it rarely causes symptoms, even while it's damaging your body. Just as with elevated cholesterol levels or high blood sugar, many women don't realize they have a problem until it becomes serious. As a physician who specializes in prevention, I find this very worrisome. Uncontrolled risk factors, such as high blood pressure, elevated cholesterol, and diabetes, significantly increase a woman's chances of both heart attack and stroke—particularly since these risk factors often occur simultaneously.

Of these risk factors, hypertension is probably the best-known.

Physicians have long recognized the negative effects high blood pressure has on the cardiovascular system, as well as other organs. However, over recent years, research has shown that these effects occur at lower levels than we previously thought, which makes it even more important to understand what high blood pressure is, how it affects our bodies, and what we can do to keep it under control.

What Is Blood Pressure?

When blood is pumped from the heart and travels through your arteries, it exerts force on the vessel walls—the amount of force is your blood pressure. The measurement consists of two numbers: the *systolic* or upper number, and the *diastolic* or lower number. The top number represents the force of your heart pumping blood into the circulatory system. As the heart rests between contractions, the pressure in the arteries lowers. The bottom number measures the lowest pressure that can be heard when the heart relaxes and refills with blood. Essentially, the numbers indicate the highest and lowest amount of blood pressure occurring within the body, which is measured in millimeters of mercury (mmHg).

The arteries respond to this pressure by contracting and expanding. Don't think of your arteries as static pipes, but rather as flexible tubes. Arteries are composed of several layers, including a fibrous outer layer,

High blood pressure (hypertension) is the most common cardiovascular risk factor. It affects more than 30 percent, or one in three adults in the United States. Left untreated, hypertension can lead to vision problems, heart attack, stroke, and other potentially fatal conditions, such as kidney failure. It is, in fact, the leading cause of stroke and a major cause of heart attack and heart failure.

a muscular layer, and a protective lining called the *endothelium*. Arteries also come in different sizes. Major arteries, which are large and can handle higher pressure, branch out into smaller and smaller vessels, ending in *arterioles*. From there, blood flows through tiny *capillaries*, which deliver oxygen where it's needed. These capillaries also remove waste, such as carbon dioxide. Even the smallest vessels play an important role in providing our organs and muscles with life-sustaining oxygen—and they are all affected by blood pressure.

How Hypertension Affects the Heart

If your blood pressure is consistently too high, the arteries adjust to withstand this increased force. Just as too much air pressure can damage a tire, too much blood pressure can damage our arteries—they respond by becoming thicker and less elastic. This thickening makes it harder for blood to flow through your arteries, and the decreased elasticity causes damage to the vessel walls. When this happens, plaque is more likely to adhere and build up (atherosclerosis), which makes the arteries stiffer and narrower. Now, a vicious cycle has begun. As the arteries become constricted and less flexible, they are unable to relax and expand properly, further increasing your blood pressure. If you smoke, which also damages the arteries and raises blood pressure, you compound the problem. So, you can see how having multiple risks factors combined with hypertension can lead to serious cardiovascular problems.

Elevated blood pressure also means your heart has to work harder. While strengthening the heart muscle through exercise is healthy, the type of muscle building that occurs within the heart to accommodate higher blood pressures is dangerous. Over time, the heart muscle begins to thicken and enlarge, making it more difficult for blood to flow into the heart and out into the arteries. This enlarging of the heart muscle is called *hypertrophy*.

Most often, we see this problem in the left ventricle, which is the main pumping chamber. Left-ventricle hypertrophy is usually a sign that a person has had hypertension for many years, and it increases a person's risk for heart attack and heart failure. Remember, if the left ventricle is not strong enough to pump blood out into the arteries, it leads to a backup of fluid in the lungs (i.e., congestive heart failure). We call this type of heart failure *diastolic heart failure*—and it is more common in women than men. In a study of almost 20,000 people treated for heart failure, about 80 percent of the patients with diastolic heart failure were women. Most likely this is due to women's tendency to develop hypertension in greater numbers as they age, and because women live longer, on average, there are more elderly women with high blood pressure.

The three major risk factors for diastolic heart failure are gender (female), age (65 years and older), and hypertension. Unfortunately, this type of heart failure is usually not recognized until symptoms are severe, which is why an early diagnosis and treatment of high blood pressure is so important. Obviously, you can't change your gender or your age, but you can keep your blood pressure in a healthy range. Symptoms of diastolic heart failure include:

- shortness of breath, often starting with activity, but possibly occurring at night when lying flat
- swelling in your feet and legs and, in some cases, your trunk or abdomen
- increase in weight
- weakness or even light-headedness

I realize these symptoms are somewhat vague, and there may be many causes for each one. For instance, a lack of regular exercise can cause shortness of breath and weight gain. Swelling in your feet and legs can sometimes be caused by an increase in activity, as well as a diet high in sodium and hormonal fluctuations. However, if you have hypertension—particularly if you have lived with it for years—and you experience one or more of these symptoms, you should consult your physician about the possibility of diastolic heart failure.

If this type of heart condition is suspected, one of the first tests to be ordered is an echocardiogram, or "echo" for short. This non-invasive test uses sound waves to take a picture of the heart as it beats. An echo will reveal the shape and thickness of the walls in the heart's chambers. It can also gauge the pressure changes in your heart, as well as the degree to which your heart relaxes between contractions. A stiff heart will need more time to relax and refill between beats.

With a diagnosis of heart failure, a physician will typically prescribe diuretics (i.e., water pills) to help the heart get rid of extra fluid, along with medications to slow the heart rate down and allow additional time between beats for the heart muscle to relax. Clearly, another very important part of the treatment is to lower blood pressure, which helps the heart to pump the blood forward into the arteries.

The Other Effects of Hypertension

In addition to heart problems, hypertension may cause many other health issues. If your arteries cannot effectively do their job of bringing oxygenated blood to your organs, these organs cannot function properly. In particular, your kidneys, which play a part in regulating blood pressure, can be severely compromised by years of hypertension. In fact, hypertension is a leading cause of kidney failure.

Hypertension is also a major risk factor for stroke. Damaged blood vessels in the brain are more likely to break open or rupture, which can cause a devastating stroke due to bleeding. Abnormal artery function can also increase the risk for embolic strokes, which are caused by small clots that become lodged in the artery and block blood flow to the brain. Many elderly women experience dementia due to multiple "attacks" or infarctions that are caused by lack of blood to the brain (similar to heart attacks) after years of living with high blood pressure.

The damaging effects of hypertension to our cardiovascular system and other organs, including our kidneys, are clear—but how high is too high?

Know Your Numbers

It was not that long ago that the medical community thought blood pressure could be quite elevated before it warranted concern. Even as late as the twentieth century, physicians believed a good goal for systolic blood pressure (the top number) was 100 plus your age. So, if you were 64 years old, your systolic blood pressure was considered "okay" up to 164 mmHg. Most physicians also considered the diastolic (or bottom number) to be the most important measurement. Now, however, we know that as we age our vessels can become stiff, which lowers the diastolic number. Consequently, it's the systolic pressure that becomes more important as we get older—a time when we are also more likely to develop hypertension. In addition, the difference between the two numbers, referred to as the *pulse pressure*, is another important gauge to determine your risk for heart disease. There are no set cutoff values for pulse pressure; care management is not changed based on this number. Rather, some people will have widened pulse pressure due to heart valve abnormalities while the majority of the population will with age and high blood pressure.

After many studies were conducted in the 1970s and 1980s, we found there was a significant reduction in the risk for cardiovascular disease with lower blood pressure, which led to earlier and more aggressive treatment. Yet, when we look at the number of adults in the United States who are aware they have high blood pressure and who are being treated effectively, the statistics have not changed much over the years. In other words, awareness has not kept up with the research. High blood pressure continues to be a growing health problem. This lack of improvement could be due to the increasing prevalence of obesity and sedentary lifestyles among American adults.

The first step in correcting this problem is awareness. It's important to know your blood pressure numbers and understand what those numbers mean (see Table 1). It amazes me to hear that even when people have their blood pressure taken during a routine exam, many don't ask what the reading is! If your health-care provider doesn't tell you what your blood pressure is, be sure to inquire. If you're told that your blood pressure is high, a repeat measurement is recommended. Patients often have slightly elevated blood pressure when they arrive at the doctor's office—maybe you were caught in traffic, or you had to rush because the sitter was

Table 1. What Your Numbers Mean (Classification of Blood Pressure for Adults)

Classification	Systolic Pressure (mmHg)	Diastolic Pressure (mmHg)
Normal	<120	and <80
Prehypertension	120–139	or 80–89
Stage 1 hypertension	140–159	or 90–99
Stage 2 hypertension	≥160	or ≥100

Source: Seventh Report of the Joint National Committee on Prevention, Detection, Evaluation, and Treatment of High Blood Pressure.

late, or you simply get anxious during medical exams. Blood pressures can vary depending on activities, emotions, or stress level.

Ideally, your blood pressure should be taken in a quiet environment, with your feet on the floor (crossing your legs can increase your blood pressure by several points) and your arm at heart level. In our clinic, if a patient's blood pressure is high, we often take three or more readings, disregarding the first reading and averaging the others.

A blood pressure reading of 140/90 mmHg or higher, taken at least twice, is considered high and warrants treatment, which includes lifestyle modifications and/or medications. A reading above 180 systolic or 100 diastolic indicates *hypertensive crisis* and requires emergency treatment.

About 50 million Americans fall into the category of prehypertension, which means they have a systolic pressure of 120–139 or a diastolic pressure of 80–89. Because the risk of heart disease increases progressively with elevated blood pressure, even these "borderline" pressures are worrisome. Prehypertension can increase your risk of cardiovascular disease more than twofold, compared to a woman whose blood pressure is under 120/80 mmHg. For every 20 mmHg increase in systolic pressure, and every 10 mmHg increase in diastolic pressure, the risk of death due to heart attack or stroke doubles. That means that a woman with a blood pressure of 145/85, for example, will have twice the risk of stroke or heart disease as compared to a woman whose blood pressure is 125/75.

Did you know? Blood pressure rises steadily from about 90/60 at birth to approximately 120/80 in a healthy adult, and tends to increase with age. It may vary from person to person and react to activities, emotion, and stress. Your blood pressure after a five-mile jog or a big presentation at work would probably be considerably higher than normal.

The good news is that, like prediabetes or slightly elevated cholesterol, prehypertension offers an opportunity to turn things around with lifestyle changes, possibly avoiding medications and the greater risk of developing hypertension. High blood pressure responds well to diet and exercise, so even if you have been diagnosed with hypertension, lifestyle changes will be very helpful in reducing or eliminating the number and dosage of medications required to get blood pressure under control.

Table 2. Recommendations for Follow-Up Based on Initial Blood Pressure Measurements*

Blood Pressure Classification	Follow-Up Recommendation
Normal	Recheck in 2 years
Prehypertension	Recheck in 1 year
Stage 1 hypertension	Confirm within 2 months
Stage 2 hypertension	Evaluate or refer to source of care within 1 month. For those with higher pressures (>180/110 mmHg), evaluate and treat immediately or within 1 week, depending on clinical situation and complications.

* For adults without acute end organ damage or other health risks.
Source: Seventh Report of the Joint National Committee on Prevention, Detection, Evaluation, and Treatment of High Blood Pressure.

Treatment for Hypertension

As mentioned, hypertension is very responsive to lifestyle changes. It goes without saying that habits such as smoking and excessive alcohol consumption should be eliminated. In addition, diet and exercise can make a huge difference. In fact, evidence suggests that even a five-pound weight loss can improve blood pressure control. Since women often tend to gain a few pounds each year during perimenopause and menopause, it's not surprising that more postmenopausal women have high blood pressure than premenopausal women. The combination of getting older and gaining weight increases your likelihood of developing high blood pressure, which makes this the perfect time to step up your activity level and improve your diet! (See chapters 11 and 12 for heart-healthy diet and exercise guidelines.)

The Sodium Link The link between sodium (salt) and high blood pressure is very strong. Though some sodium is essential to our bodies for fluid balance, muscle strength, and nerve function, most people get far too much salt from their diets. The U.S. Department of Health and Human Services dietary guidelines call for less than 2,300 milligrams per day (about 1 teaspoon); however, older adults, African-Americans, and those with a diagnosis of hypertension should only be consuming 1,500 milligrams. Unfortunately, it's estimated that most Americans get double or even triple those amounts each day! It's no wonder we have such high rates of hypertension.

Many of my patients tell me they are not using the saltshaker at home and are still not seeing an improvement in their blood pressure. That's because 80 percent of our salt intake comes from sodium in processed foods—not what we add with the saltshaker.

Who Is at Risk for Developing Hypertension?

While anyone can have high blood pressure (including children and teens), there are some factors that put you at a higher risk. You may be more likely to develop hypertension if you:

- have a family history of high blood pressure
- are African-American
- are over age 55
- are overweight
- are not physically active
- drink excessively
- smoke
- eat foods high in saturated fats and sodium
- take certain medications such as NSAIDs (ibuprofen, aspirin, etc.), decongestants, or use illegal drugs

At 63, Maureen is recently retired and enjoying her role as a grandparent. When she gets together with her friends, they share photos and stories of their grandchildren, as well as a couple of cigarettes. Since she is only a "social smoker," Maureen has never been concerned about quitting. She doesn't exercise regularly, but considers chasing after her two-year-old granddaughter and golfing with her husband plenty of activity. She sometimes feels fatigued and would like to lose a few pounds, but overall, she believes her health is good.

One day, while shopping with her daughter, who is expecting her second child, they noticed one of those blood pressure machines at the pharmacy. Maureen's daughter, who is very health conscious, urged her mother to check her blood pressure. Since it had been years since she had her blood pressure checked, she thought "what the heck"—and was very surprised by the reading! At 149/90, she was considered hypertensive. Concerned, Maureen made an appointment with her physician.

After taking her blood pressure several times, the doctor confirmed the diagnosis. He gave Maureen some medication to help lower her blood pressure, along with information on a low-sodium diet. Though reluctant to take any medication, she agreed to fill the prescription when the doctor outlined the increased cardiovascular risks associated with hypertension. He reminded her, however, that with lifestyle changes (i.e., diet and exercise) she might be able to lower her blood pressure and eventually discontinue the medications. That was motivating for Maureen, who loves a good challenge.

She began reading food labels and was amazed by the amount of sodium in many of the foods she ate regularly. Much to her husband's dismay, she removed the saltshaker from the table and bought a heart-healthy cookbook. In the beginning, both Maureen and her husband found the lack of sodium difficult—foods tasted bland. However, as time went on and Maureen began experimenting with herbs and spices, they began to really enjoy the taste of their meals. In fact, when she ordered her favorite French onion soup at a local restaurant, she found it overly salty.

Maureen dreaded the idea of daily exercise, but she found a neighbor who was interested in walking with her every morning. As the two women walked and talked, this daily ritual became something to which they both looked forward. Of course, the last piece of the puzzle was giving up the occasional cigarettes. When she informed her friends about her hypertension, she found they were very supportive, and eventually she was able to quit smoking for good.

At her six-month checkup, both Maureen and her doctor were pleasantly surprised by her blood pressure reading, which was near normal. He told her that if she maintained these lifestyle changes and kept her blood pressure down, she could try discontinuing the medication. Maureen had to admit that she had more energy and felt better than she had in years. She had assumed that her lack of energy was simply due to getting older. And having more energy was going to come in handy with the birth of her second grandchild!

We have grown up eating these foods and, because our taste buds have become accustomed to the flavor, they don't taste salty to us. Lowering your sodium consumption often means reorienting your taste buds to foods without added salt. Cooking at home, using herbs and spices instead of salt, and eliminating hidden sources of sodium (see The Salty Dozen, page 91) will open your palate to a whole new world of healthy options that taste great.

I tell my patients to read nutrition labels and become aware of which foods contain high levels of sodium, as well as saturated fats and cholesterol. Many good smartphone and computer apps also allow you to enter foods and review the amount of salt you consume each day. If you do this periodically, you might be surprised by how quickly the sodium adds up! You can even make it a family contest. Data suggest that children and young adults are getting too much salt in their diets, setting them up for future health problems; so the earlier you get them involved and educated the better.

Medications Though diet and exercise are very effective, many women with hypertension will also need to take medications to control their blood pressure. I understand that some people are reluctant to take medications, which may have side effects, but when you consider the risk for stroke, heart attacks, and even kidney failure that come along with hypertension, using medication to lower blood pressure can be lifesaving. I counsel my patients on the importance of taking medications along with lifestyle modifications. If they are able to significantly change their lifestyles and keep those changes in place for a substantial period of time, then they are often able to reduce or eliminate medications.

Many types of medications are used to lower blood pressure, giving you and your health-care provider a wide range of options to find one that works for your individual needs. The most common drugs used to treat hypertension include:

DASH to the Rescue

A major study called DASH (Dietary Approaches to Stop Hypertension) demonstrated the benefits of healthy eating on blood pressure reduction. The study focused on a diet high in fruits and vegetables, along with low-fat dairy products. Whole grains were encouraged, along with a reduction in foods high in saturated fats. Even though the amount of sodium allowed in the diet was higher than our current recommendations, the participants significantly lowered their blood pressures. DASH participants who were classified as prehypertensive (120–139 mmHg) reduced their systolic blood pressure an average of 6 mmHg, while those with hypertension (140 mmHg or higher) lowered their systolic pressure an average of 11 mmHg—and started seeing results in as little as two weeks! A second study examined lower sodium intake along with the DASH eating plan (about 1,500 mg/day, or 2/3 of a teaspoon). This group saw the largest reductions in blood pressure—both systolic and diastolic.

For more information and recipes visit www.dashdiet.org

- Beta-blockers, which control the rate and strength of the heart's contractions
- Calcium-channel blockers, which decrease blood pressure by changing an electrical signal so the heart does not contract so strongly
- ACE inhibitors, which work on the kidneys instead of the heart
- Diuretics, which help the body rid itself of excess fluid, reducing pressure on blood vessel walls.

Based on your overall health and blood pressure goals, your physician will prescribe one or more of these medications. Some people respond better to one type of medication than another. It often takes some trial and error to discover the best treatment for you, so be patient.

Low Blood Pressure It is possible to lower blood pressure too much. If your blood pressure is too low, organs such as your brain are not receiving an adequate amount of blood, which can cause light-headedness and, in some cases, fainting. Because low blood pressure can be dangerous, it's important to work closely with your physician to monitor your medications and recheck your blood pressure regularly. Controlling hypertension is a partnership between you and your physician.

Take a Step

Since hypertension is such a significant risk factor for heart disease—and because blood pressure tends to increase as we age—early prevention is the best treatment. To keep your blood pressure in a healthy range, take these simple steps:

- Get Tested—Be sure to have your blood pressure checked regularly. If it's normal, you can prevent future problems with a healthy diet and exercise. If it's borderline or prehypertensive, you can make lifestyle modifications, such as reducing sodium and saturated fats in your diet and increasing your activity level. If it's high, talk to your physician about medication, along with lifestyle changes. Remember, hypertension can be effectively treated, and every small drop in blood pressure significantly reduces your risk of cardiovascular problems!
- Get Motivated

Be a label reader—Watch for hidden sodium (as well as saturated fats) in the foods you regularly eat. Look for low-sodium or no-salt added versions of your favorite foods.

Cook at home—When you prepare more meals at home instead of relying on fast food or take out, you can control the amount of sodium and fat, which is often "off the charts" in restaurants.

Step up your activity—Exercising regularly can not only improve your blood pressure, but also reduce your cholesterol levels and help you lose weight. Even a five-pound weight loss can lower your blood pressure.

The Salty Dozen

Aside from the obvious culprits—salty snacks such as chips and pretzels—sodium is often hidden in seemingly innocent foods. Some of the worst offenders include:

1. **Frozen dinners**—These quick and easy options are often loaded with sodium. Don't be fooled by "lighter" versions, which may have less fat and calories, but are still high in salt.

2. **Ready-to-eat cereals**—It may surprise you to find that some brands have up to 250 milligrams of sodium per cup. Read labels carefully.

3. **Vegetable juices**—These may seem like a good way to get your daily servings of veggies, but look out: some have up to 479 mg of sodium per cup. Look for low-sodium versions.

4. **Canned vegetables**—The preservatives and sauces used in canned veggies often add extra salt—up to 730 mg per cup! You can rinse the vegetables before cooking or look for no-salt-added versions.

5. **Packaged deli meats**—Some have more sodium than others, so read labels carefully. If you buy your lunch meat at the deli counter, you can ask for low-sodium brands.

6. **Soups**—You might be shocked to find that your favorite brand of chicken noodle soup has 744 mg of sodium in every cup. Look for reduced sodium versions or, better yet, make homemade soup.

7. **Marinades and flavorings**—One tablespoon of teriyaki sauce has 690 mg of sodium, and one tablespoon of soy sauce has 1,024 mg! Even low-sodium varieties are high in salt. Use them sparingly or try marinating meats in vinegar, lemon juice, and other fruit juices, such as orange and pineapple.

8. **Spaghetti sauce**—Popular brands contain 500–600 mg of sodium per ½ cup. Again, look for no-salt-added versions, or try making sauce from scratch using pepper, oregano, basil, and sodium-free spice blends for flavor.

9. **Nuts**—Salt content varies widely by brand, so look for unsalted or low-sodium versions.

10. **Prepackaged rice, potatoes, and pasta**—On their own, rice, potatoes, and pasta have very little to no sodium, but when they are packaged with seasonings and sauces, they can be loaded with salt. Read labels carefully or prepare your own.

11. **Condiments**—Ketchup, relish, capers, and other condiments can pack a wallop when it comes to sodium. Read labels and watch serving sizes.

12. **Prepared spice blends**—Steak rubs, Asian blends, and other flavored seasonings often contain salt as a main ingredient. There are many no-salt or low-sodium spice blends available, such as the Mrs. Dash varieties. (One note: women with kidney problems should watch the level of potassium in some of these spice blends.)

Source: Based on a list compiled by WebMD, 2012

CHAPTER SEVEN

The Cholesterol Connection

Follow your heart, but take your brain with you.

UNKNOWN

We hear a lot about cholesterol. Just recently, while waiting in line at the grocery store, I noticed several magazines featuring low-cholesterol diets and recipes. There is an entire shelf of books devoted to managing cholesterol at our local bookstore, and nightly television commercials advertise a number of cholesterol-lowering drugs. It seems that every day we learn about a natural supplement or miracle food that promises to reduce cholesterol. Since the link between cholesterol and heart health is very strong, I'm glad the message is getting out. Yet, despite all the available information, there still seems to be some confusion. What does it really mean to have healthy cholesterol levels? What is the difference between "good" and "bad" cholesterol, and how do you translate all those numbers? Once you have a basic understanding of what cholesterol is and how it affects our bodies, both positively and negatively, you can begin to make better choices to improve your heart health.

What Is Cholesterol?

Cholesterol is a waxy, fatlike substance or lipid. Lipid is just another name for fat, derived from the Greek word *lipos*, meaning "fat." Made primarily in the liver, cholesterol is necessary for our bodies to function properly. In fact, cholesterol is used to produce hormones, vitamin D, and digestive enzymes. It also plays an important role in nerve and brain health. However, as with glucose and other natural substances in your body, you can have too much of a good thing.

In a healthy system, the liver only produces as much cholesterol as the body needs. We also acquire cholesterol from the foods we eat. According to the American Heart Association, about 25 percent of the cholesterol found in our bodies comes from food sources. Animal-based foods that contain saturated fats, such as meats and eggs, as well as processed foods that contain trans fats, are converted into cholesterol in the body. In addition to diet, many other factors may affect your cholesterol level, including:

- **Weight**—Being overweight can increase your cholesterol. Conversely, losing weight can reduce the amount of total cholesterol in your body, while raising levels of good cholesterol. In general, the more body fat you have, the more cholesterol you will have.
- **Exercise**—Regular exercise (at least 30 minutes on most days) can lower your total cholesterol levels by decreasing bad cholesterol while increasing the amount of good cholesterol in the body. (We will discuss the difference between good and bad cholesterol in the following pages.)
- **Heredity**—Your genes partly determine how much cholesterol your body manufactures. If your parent(s) had high cholesterol, you may be more likely to have high cholesterol.

In addition, inherited defects in the cholesterol pathway can cause very high cholesterol in some people. If these elevated cholesterol levels include too much bad cholesterol, these individuals have an increased risk for heart disease at a younger age—as early as their twenties. These patients often need to be seen in a specialized lipid clinic and require medication to help manage their cholesterol, even when they are children. There are also certain genetic disorders that cause abnormally high cholesterol levels. For most of us, however, cholesterol can be effectively controlled with lifestyle modifications.

- **Gender**—Before menopause, women tend to have lower cholesterol levels than men of the same age. However, after menopause, the level of bad cholesterol in women tends to rise, putting them at a higher risk for heart disease.
- **Age**—Cholesterol levels typically increase as we get older.
- **Smoking**—As we will learn in chapter 9, smoking not only decreases good cholesterol, it worsens the effects of bad cholesterol by making the arterial walls more receptive to plaque buildup.
- **Stress**—Studies show that increased levels of mental and emotional stress over long periods of time can raise your cholesterol and make it more destructive.
- **Other causes**—Certain medications and medical conditions can cause high cholesterol. There are also medications (statins) used to reduce cholesterol in the body.

While there are some things you can't change, such as your genes, your gender, or your age, you can improve your cholesterol levels through diet, exercise, stress reduction, and not smoking. However, total cholesterol levels do not tell the complete story. To understand the effects of cholesterol on our hearts, we need to know about the different types of cholesterol and how they work within our bodies.

The Good, the Bad, and the Triglycerides

Often, when a woman comes to my medical practice, she has been told that her total cholesterol is elevated, which puts her at a higher risk for cardiovascular problems. Determining your total cholesterol is an important first step, but it's not enough. To make an accurate assessment, we need to look at your complete "cholesterol profile," which includes measuring the different types of cholesterol found in the bloodstream. In order for cholesterol, which is waxy, to travel through the blood, which is watery, it receives a coating of protein. These cholesterol-protein bundles are called *lipoproteins*. Each type of lipoprotein has a specific function.

- **High-density lipoproteins (HDL)**—HDL is often called "good" cholesterol because its main job is to pick up excess fat in the bloodstream and carry it back to the liver for processing or metabolizing. By removing this excess fat from your arteries, HDL helps reduce plaque formation. So, having higher levels of HDL in your cholesterol profile may lower your risk for cardiovascular disease. (I tell my patients to think of the "H" in HDL as "higher.")
- **Low-density lipoproteins (LDL)**—As with HDL, the function of LDL is to transport cholesterol through your blood, but unlike HDL, it mainly delivers the cholesterol to your arteries. Everyone needs some cholesterol, including LDL cholesterol, but we know that when LDL cholesterol levels are high it begins to accumulate on artery walls and form atherosclerotic plaque. While it's known as the "bad"

cholesterol, it's only bad when there is too much in your bloodstream. Elevated LDL levels increase your risk for cardiovascular problems. Therefore, the primary goal of therapy is lowering LDL cholesterol, which we know from many studies significantly reduces your risk of heart attacks and stroke.

- **Triglycerides**—Triglycerides are another type of fat carried in your bloodstream. They are made up of fatty acids along with a sticky substance called glycerol. Like HDL and LDL cholesterol, triglycerides are made in our body and found in the foods we eat. They are stored in our fat cells and provide a great way for the body to stockpile fuel for future needs. However, in our modern culture, we typically don't experience times of famine when these fat stores become necessary. Therefore, we often end up with excess triglycerides. And it's not just fatty foods that are converted into triglycerides. If we consume more calories in a meal than our bodies require, we can raise our triglyceride levels. Researchers at Harvard found that women who had elevated triglycerides after they ate were at a higher risk for heart disease. Also, if the triglyceride levels are very high, other problems such as pancreatitis (a painful inflammation of the pancreas) are more likely to develop.

If a woman has elevated triglycerides it's important to review her medications, including any supplements she may be taking. Sometimes medications such as oral contraceptives can raise triglycerides. Additionally, when I see a patient with elevated triglycerides, I look closely for the presence of diabetes or prediabetes. Many women (and men) with poor glucose control will have high triglycerides and lower HDL cholesterol as well. In general, women tend to have higher triglyceride levels than men.

If there are more triglycerides in the bloodstream than your body needs, the surplus can build up on the walls of arteries, contributing to heart disease.

The link between high cholesterol and heart health is powerful. Data from the Second National Health and Nutrition Examination Survey showed that 55 percent of women who died from coronary heart disease had a total cholesterol level of 240 mg/dL, which is considered very high.

One of the reasons heart disease is so prevalent in the United States is that a large number of both men and women in our country have cholesterol levels that are too high. An estimated 16.2 percent or 33 million adults living in the United States have total cholesterol levels of 240 mg/dL or greater, which puts them at increased risk for cardiovascular disease. Even more worrisome is that much of this is due to elevated levels of LDL or bad cholesterol.

Why do so many people have high cholesterol? Put simply, we eat too many fatty foods and we don't get enough exercise! More and more, we are seeing the effects of these lifestyle factors in children and young adults who are already developing unhealthy cholesterol profiles. This translates into higher levels of bad cholesterol and lower levels of good cholesterol starting from an early age. Since we know that it takes time for atherosclerosis to develop and cause problems, you can see that unhealthy cholesterol profiles at an early age lead to heart disease in younger people. As a result, we are finding a greater number of young women with cardiovascular problems—we now see women having heart attacks in their 40s rather than at age 60 or 70. Many of these women have high cholesterol together with other cardiac risk factors, such as smoking, high blood pressure, or diabetes.

How Cholesterol Affects the Heart

The connection between high cholesterol and heart disease is undeniable: one study found that over half of individuals who died from heart disease had total cholesterol levels of 240 mg/dL or greater. Our bodies were not made to process this much cholesterol. As we learned, there is a delicate balance between the amount of cholesterol the body needs and the amount we manufacture and consume. When this balance is disrupted, our systems become overloaded and begin to break down. Several things can happen: (1) we may have more LDLs than the body requires; (2) the liver does not produce or release enough HDLs to pick up the excess; or (3) the liver does not correctly signal to the body when cholesterol is too high. Often, the liver gets bogged down with fatty deposits and does not work effectively.

In each case, the excess LDL cholesterol begins to build up on the walls of our arteries. If the arterial walls are already compromised due to other risk factors, such as high blood pressure, diabetes, or smoking, then this buildup is more likely to occur. Over time, the plaque begins to harden, blocking the flow of blood and oxygen to our hearts and brains, which may lead to a heart attack or stroke. Plaque may also become unstable and break open, leading to a heart attack even if the plaque is not very large.

As we discussed in chapter 5, "Assessing Your Risk," cholesterol is only one of the risk factors associated with cardiovascular disease. Obviously, having more than one risk factor increases your chances of developing problems. Having high cholesterol along with hypertension (high blood pressure) or diabetes, for instance, can be a dangerous combination when it comes to heart health. That's why we look at a woman's overall health when we discuss cholesterol levels and possible treatments.

Know Your Numbers

Everyone should have their cholesterol levels tested regularly—and know what the numbers mean (see Table 3). Current guidelines recommend cholesterol screening beginning at the age of 20, and then tests every five years—unless you have elevated cholesterol levels or other health issues, in which case you need to be tested more frequently. Although the number of adults who report having their cholesterol checked has increased from 68.6 percent to 74.8 percent over the last ten years, many people are still unaware of their cholesterol levels. Women and minorities, in particular, remain less informed about their cholesterol numbers compared to men and non-minorities. Reduced access to screening and medical care may account for these differences. Even among those people who have high cholesterol and meet the criteria for drug therapy, many are not receiving proper treatment.

The first step is to get tested. Cholesterol screening consists of a simple blood test, which is done after fasting for 9 to 12 hours. By not eating or drinking prior to the test, you obtain more accurate information regarding your LDL and triglyceride levels. Certain foods and beverages, particularly alcohol, will cause your profile to change, especially triglyceride levels. You can interpret the results of your cholesterol screening as follows:

- With HDL (good) cholesterol, higher levels are better. Low HDL cholesterol (less than 40 mg/dL for men, less than 50 mg/dL for women) puts you at higher risk for heart disease. In the average man, HDL cholesterol levels range from 40 to 50 mg/dL. In the average woman, they range from 50 to 60 mg/dL.
- HDL cholesterol of 60 mg/dL or higher gives some protection against heart disease. The mean level of HDL choles-

Table 3. Interpreting Cholesterol Test Results

Total Cholesterol Level	Category
Less than 200 mg/dL	A desirable level that puts you at lower risk for coronary heart disease. A cholesterol level of 200 mg/dL or higher raises your risk.
200–239 mg/dL	Borderline high
240 mg/dL and above	High blood cholesterol. A person with this level has more than twice the risk of coronary heart disease of someone whose cholesterol is below 200 mg/dL.
HDL Cholesterol Level	**Category**
Less than 40 mg/dL (for men) Less than 50 mg/dL (for women)	Low HDL cholesterol. A major risk factor for heart disease.
60 mg/dL and above	High HDL cholesterol. An HDL of 60 mg/dL and above is considered protective against heart disease.
LDL Cholesterol Level	**Category**
Less than 100 mg/dL	Optimal
100–129 mg/dL	Near or above optimal
130–159 mg/dL	Borderline high
160–189 mg/dL	High
190 mg/dL and above	Very high
Triglyceride Level	**Category**
Less than 150 mg/dL	Normal
150–199 mg/dL	Borderline high
200–499 mg/dL	High
500 mg/dL and above	Very high

terol for American adults age 20 and older is 54.3 mg/dL.

- Smoking, being overweight, and being sedentary can all result in lower HDL cholesterol. To raise your HDL level, avoid tobacco smoke, maintain a healthy weight, and get at least 30 to 60 minutes of physical activity more days than not.
- People with high blood triglycerides usually also have lower HDL cholesterol and a higher risk of heart attack and stroke. Progesterone, anabolic steroids, and male sex hormones (testosterone) also lower HDL cholesterol levels. Female sex hormones raise HDL cholesterol levels.
- The lower your LDL cholesterol, the lower your risk of heart attack and stroke. In fact, it's a better gauge of risk than total blood cholesterol. Your other risk factors for heart disease and stroke help determine what your LDL level should be, as well as the appropriate treatment for you. A healthy level for you may not be healthy for your friend or neighbor. Discuss your levels and your treatment options with your doctor to get the plan that works for you. The mean level of LDL cholesterol for American adults age 20 and older is 115.0 mg/dL.
- Triglycerides are the most common type of fat in the body. Many people who have heart disease or diabetes have high triglyceride levels. Normal triglyceride levels vary by age and sex. A high triglyceride level combined with low HDL cholesterol or high LDL cholesterol seems to speed up atherosclerosis (the buildup of fatty deposits in artery walls). Atherosclerosis increases the risk for heart attack and stroke.
- Many people have high triglyceride levels due to being overweight/obese, physical inactivity, cigarette smoking,

excess alcohol consumption, and/or a diet very high in carbohydrates (60 percent or more of calories). High triglycerides are a lifestyle-related risk factor, but underlying diseases or genetic disorders may be the cause. The mean level of triglycerides for American adults age 20 and older is 144.2 mg/dL.

- The main therapy to reduce triglyceride levels is to change your lifestyle. This means control your weight, eat a heart-healthy diet, get regular physical activity, avoid tobacco smoke, limit alcohol to one drink per day for women or two drinks per day for men, and limit beverages and foods with added sugars. Visit your health-care provider to create an action plan that will incorporate all these lifestyle changes. Sometimes, medication is needed in addition to a healthy diet and lifestyle.

- A triglyceride level of 150 mg/dL or higher is one of the risk factors of metabolic syndrome. Metabolic syndrome increases the risk for heart disease and other disorders, including diabetes.

For more information on when to get tested, visit www.heart.org and search "how to get your cholesterol tested."

When to Consider Medication

Most people can prevent high cholesterol with a healthy diet and regular exercise, along with routine checkups. The need for cholesterol-lowering medications is more common in middle-aged and older adults, or those who have been unsuccessful at reducing levels with lifestyle changes. Sometimes patients will ask me if they should begin taking a cholesterol-lowering medication because a friend or neighbor who has the same cholesterol level is on one. But the decision to prescribe a medication is not based solely on cholesterol levels. We need to consider a woman's overall health, including other cardiovascular risk factors.

Health-care professionals are primarily concerned with LDL or bad cholesterol. When a person has a heart attack, one of the first things most physicians do is prescribe a medication to lower LDL cholesterol. The reason for the focus on LDL cholesterol is that multiple studies have shown that both men and women with high LDL levels are at an increased risk for atherosclerosis, and thus heart attacks and strokes. These studies have also demonstrated that lowering LDL cholesterol with medication can reduce a person's risk for cardiovascular disease between 25 and 40 percent.

The target range for LDL levels depends on other risk factors. For example, women with coronary artery disease (CAD), or who are at risk of developing CAD, should aim for an LDL level under 70 mg/dL. Women who have diabetes should target an LDL level of less than 100 mg/dL. On the other hand, a woman with no other cardiac risk factors may be fine with slightly higher LDL levels. This is why guidelines from the American Heart Association and other medical societies have different LDL goals. In general, the higher a woman's risk, the more beneficial a cholesterol-lowering medication or statins become. It's important to work with your health-care provider and consider all your risk factors when developing a treatment plan.

Table 4 provides a detailed look at LDL goals for various risk factors, as well as the levels that may warrant drug therapy versus lifestyle changes. For more information on LDL targets for patients with other risk factors, go to www.nhlbi.nih.gov/guidelines/cholesterol/atglance.htm. (See chapter 5, "Assessing Your Risk," to determine your risk category.)

Table 4. LDL Goals Based on Risk Factors

Risk Category	LDL Goal	LDL Level at Which to Initiate Therapeutic Lifestyle Changes	LDL Level at Which to Consider Drug Therapy
Has been diagnosed with CHD or has CHD Risk Equivalents* (10-year risk >20%)	<100 mg/dL	≥100 mg/dL	≥130 mg/dL (100–129 mg/dL: drug optional)**
2+ risk factors (10-year risk ≤20%)	<130 mg/dL	≥130 mg/dL	10-year risk 10–20%: ≥130 mg/dL 10-year risk <10%: ≥160 mg/dL
0–1 risk factor	<160 mg/dL	≥160 mg/dL	≥190 mg/dL (160–189 mg/dL: LDL-lowering drug optional)

* CHD risk equivalents include diabetes, carotid artery disease, peripheral artery disease, and having multiple risk factors. Major risk factors include smoking, high blood pressure, low HDL cholesterol, a family history of premature heart disease, and age.
** Some authorities recommend use of LDL-lowering drugs in this category if an LDL cholesterol <100 mg/dL cannot be achieved by therapeutic lifestyle changes. Others prefer use of drugs that primarily modify triglycerides and HDL.

Treatment Options

The primary medications used to reduce LDL cholesterol are called statins (or HMG CoA reductase inhibitors). Statins reduce the formation of cholesterol in the liver by blocking an enzyme used to make LDL cholesterol. While these medications are very good at reducing LDL or bad cholesterol, and therefore lowering the risk for heart attacks, some statins work better than others. There are many types of statins, including lovastatin, simvastin, pravastin, fluvastin, and atorvastin, which are marketed under different brand names. Deciding on a particular statin depends on your individual health condition and LDL goals. Your health-care provider can help you determine which statin and dosage are right for you.

In general, statins are very safe. The number of people who have serious side effects is extremely low. Some patients will complain of achy muscles while taking statins. As a physician, it's often difficult to tell if the statin is causing the problem, or if the patient is experiencing general aches and pains due to physical activity or arthritis. Serious muscle problems are rare, but if you experience muscle pain while taking a statin, you should consult your doctor right away. Prescribing a different statin or changing the dosage may alleviate the problem. All prescription medications, including statins, should be taken only under the guidance of a physician.

Keep in mind, statin therapy does not replace a healthy lifestyle! Medication simply complements any changes you make to your diet and exercise habits. Like most medications, statins are more effective when used in conjunction with lifestyle modifications. Patients who take statins along with adopting healthy habits are able to significantly improve their cholesterol profile and reduce their risk of cardiovascular disease.

In addition to statins, other available medications help reduce the amount of cholesterol your body absorbs or increase the amount of cholesterol your body gets rid of. In addition, plant stanols/sterols (natural supplements) can aid in the reduction of LDL cholesterol and are widely available. If your LDL levels are only slightly elevated and you are at a low risk for heart disease, this may be a better option for you.

Statins work primarily to reduce LDL cholesterol (although modest improvements in HDL and triglyceride levels may be observed). So, is there a medication that effectively increases HDL or good cholesterol? For years we have used niacin to help raise HDL. However, although niacin can improve HDL, there is no strong evidence that heart attacks and strokes are prevented.

There is currently a great deal of research being conducted on HDL cholesterol, and it's likely that new therapies will be developed in the future. In the meantime, lifestyle factors are the best way to raise HDL levels and protect your heart. I have seen some of my patients increase their HDL levels significantly by exercising regularly. This increase may be due in part to a change in weight. Weight loss, particularly around the waistline, can boost HDL cholesterol. Conversely, when a woman gains weight around her middle, she will often see a decrease in her HDL levels.

In the peri- and post-menopause years, women tend to gain weight around the waist. This type of weight gain is associated with lower levels of HDL cholesterol, so it's not surprising to see HDL levels decrease during these years—putting women at greater risk of cardiovascular problems. Of course, this makes it the perfect time to revamp your lifestyle. A healthy diet and regular exercise can not only help you get your waistline back; it can also significantly increase heart-healthy HDL cholesterol.

What about triglycerides? While statins do not often significantly decrease triglycerides, they are very responsive to dietary changes—especially a reduction in certain types of fats and carbohydrates. (We will talk more about the heart-healthy diet in chapter 11, "Eating for Life.")

When lifestyle changes are not enough and triglycerides remain very high, medications such as fibrates (or fibric acid) are sometimes prescribed. However, fibrates are not effective in lowering LDL cholesterol, so your physician may consider combining a fibrate with a statin, if necessary. In addition, natural supplements, such as fish oil, ground flaxseeds, and flaxseed oil, can help get your triglycerides in a healthy range. If you have elevated triglycerides, working with a registered dietician or nutritionist can also be very beneficial.

Take a Step

Managing your cholesterol levels can reduce your chances of developing cardiovascular problems. For most people, cholesterol can be kept in check with positive lifestyle changes, including a heart-healthy diet and regular exercise. Get started today with these simple steps:

- Get Tested—Cholesterol screening involves a simple fasting blood test. Once you know your numbers, you can begin to manage them effectively. If your cholesterol profile (HDL, LDL and triglyceride level) is within a healthy range, congratulations! Keep up the good work. If your LDL and triglycerides are slightly elevated and your HDL is lower than it should be, now is the time to make some positive lifestyle changes. If your numbers put you in a high-risk category, talk to your physician about statin therapy, along with lifestyle modifications.

- Get Motivated
  Exercising regularly (at least 30 minutes per day on most days) can boost heart-healthy HDL levels, while lowering LDL and triglyceride levels. Start a daily walking routine, join an exercise class, or get the family involved in a regular sport. An evening bike ride or a game of tennis is a great way to spend time with the family and boost your heart health! The more you do, the better the HDL-raising response you will have.

- Make a Swap
  Simple changes in your diet can go a long way toward lowering your total cholesterol. Replace refined carbs (such as white flour and rice) with whole grains. Add more fresh fruits and vegetables to your meals, and trade full-fat dairy products for fat-free or 1 percent options. Stick to lean proteins and consider meatless meals—having fish or a vegetarian dish even one night a week can make a big difference. (Turn to chapter 11, "Eating for Life," for more dietary tips.)

CHAPTER EIGHT

Diabetes and Your Heart

To me, the only things of interest are those linked to the heart.

AUDREY HEPBURN

Medical science teaches us that everything is linked; illnesses in one area of the body often lead to problems in other parts of our anatomy. We've already learned that clogged arteries can cause a number of health issues, including heart disease, and that there are many risk factors connected to our hearts (see chapter 5, "Assessing Your Risk"). Of these, diabetes is one of the strongest risk factors for cardiovascular disease a woman can have. Women who have diabetes are three to seven times more likely to develop heart disease than those without diabetes.

Unfortunately, a large number of women are affected by diabetes—an estimated 8 million in the United States—and that number is rising. This increase is directly related to the growing problem of obesity in our country. However, even if a woman is not considered obese, accumulating excess fat around the waistline can increase her chance of developing diabetes. In addition, women of color, including Asian, African-American, and Native American women have a higher risk for diabetes.

Of course, it's not just women who are at risk. Approximately 9 percent of all Americans have type 2 diabetes, or diabetes mellitus. However, only 64 percent of these people are aware they have the disorder. That means that over 25 percent, or one in four, people with diabetes don't even know they have a chronic condition that puts them at greater risk for heart disease, stroke, and even kidney failure! Equally worrisome is the fact that among those who have been properly diagnosed with diabetes, fewer than 25 percent have their condition under control. In other words, more than three out of four adults with diabetes have poorly controlled blood glucose levels and are putting their health in serious danger.

Medical researchers are not sure why, but women with diabetes are at a greater risk of heart disease than men with diabetes. Women who have diabetes are three to seven times more likely to develop problems with the heart, versus two to three times for men, according to the American Heart Association. Therefore, it's very important for women to have their blood sugar tested, and treat diabetes early and aggressively to avoid future complications.

What Is Diabetes?

Despite the recent popularity of many zero- or low-carb diets, carbohydrates are not necessarily bad. In fact, complex carbohydrates, such as whole grain cereals, breads, fruits, and vegetables, provide an important source of energy for our bodies, as well as fiber and other nutrients. On the other hand, simple carbohydrates, most readily found in candy, bakery goods, or soda, provide no essential nutrients and do more harm than good. When we eat foods high in carbohydrates, our bodies break these carbs down into glucose, which is also referred to as blood sugar. We need glucose for energy, and a healthy system is able to efficiently convert this glucose into fuel for our bodies.

The star of this conversion process is the pancreas. The pancreas produces and releases insulin into the bloodstream. Insulin is a hormone that takes glucose from the blood and stores it in the liver, muscles, and fat tissues for later use as energy. Basically, it helps regulate our metabolism and allows our cells to use glucose as fuel. Unless there is a problem, insulin is provided within the body in a constant proportion to the amount of glucose in the bloodstream, which otherwise would be toxic. When you have diabetes, either the pancreas is incapable of producing insulin or the insulin it produces is inadequate and cannot be used properly.

There are two types of diabetes: type 1 and type 2. Type 1 diabetes is an autoimmune condition that typically occurs in children and young adults. In the past, you may have heard this condition referred to as juvenile diabetes or insulin-dependent diabetes. For reasons that are still unknown, the immune system of those with type 1 diabetes begins to attack the pancreas, and eventually the organ becomes impaired and unable to produce insulin. Since the pancreas produces no insulin, those with type 1 diabetes require daily insulin injections. Though diet and exercise can help a person control the condition, lifestyle modifications cannot reverse it. Although children and young adults are unlikely to have heart disease, individuals with type 1 diabetes are still at greater risk for developing heart problems as they age, particularly if they do not control the condition properly.

The majority of people with diabetes (90 to 95 percent) have type 2, which is a metabolic disorder. With type 2, the pancreas produces some insulin, but not enough to allow the glucose to enter the body's cells. In addition, the cells develop a resistance to the insulin. Although scientists have yet to identify the exact cause of this insulin resistance, evidence indicates that it's related to excess body fat, especially belly fat.

If left untreated or not controlled properly, diabetes can have many negative effects on the body. In addition to an increased risk for heart disease and stroke, diabetes can lead to problems with the kidneys and liver. Because those with diabetes have high levels of glucose in their bloodstreams, the kidneys have to work extra hard to filter the blood and remove the excess glucose. This causes frequent urination and excessive thirst, which are two important warning signs of diabetes. Over time, this demand on the kidneys can lead to kidney disease or kidney failure. Similarly, the liver, which also helps the body maintain normal blood sugar levels and stores glucose for fuel, has to work harder than normal when there are elevated levels of glucose in the bloodstream.

Diabetes can also cause *neuropathy*, or nerve damage, which causes areas of the body to be less sensitive—often the legs and feet. In addition, diabetes impairs the body's ability to heal efficiently due to decreased blood flow. This is a dangerous combination: if you have less sensation in your feet, you may not notice a cut or scrape, and because your body is unable to heal properly, even a minor wound is more likely to get infected. If the neuropathy affects the optic nerve (the area of the eye that gives us sight), a person with diabetes may experience vision problems and, eventually, blindness. Even common illnesses, such as influenza and pneumonia, can pose serious complications for those with diabetes. When you consider all of these potential problems, you begin to understand the life-threatening nature of this disorder. In fact, diabetes is the one of the top ten causes of death in the United States.

How Diabetes Affects the Heart

Diabetes can affect the heart in two ways. First, a consistently high level of blood sugar causes damage to the arteries, allowing plaque to adhere and accumulate more easily. In other words, it makes atherosclerosis more likely to develop. As we know, this leads to decreased blood flow to the heart and possibly the brain, increasing your chances of heart attack and stroke. Secondly, diabetes can make the heart require more blood flow, forcing it to work harder.

The connection between heart health and diabetes is very strong—about two-thirds of those with diabetes die from cardio-vascular disease. And, this bears repeating, women with diabetes are at a higher risk for heart disease than men. In fact, women with diabetes are at the same risk for a future heart attack as a woman who has already had a heart attack; and women with both heart disease and diabetes are at the highest risk for lethal heart events. While we don't know why diabetes is particularly deadly among women, we do know how to prevent diabetes, as well as detect and treat it effectively.

The Warning Signs

As with high blood pressure and high cholesterol, the best treatment for diabetes is prevention. However, if you do develop diabetes, early detection and treatment can help you avoid complications and protect your heart. Consequently, it's important to know the signs and symptoms of this condition, which may include:

- frequent urination
- excessive thirst
- extreme hunger
- unusual weight loss

- increased fatigue
- irritability (caused by fluctuations in blood sugar)
- numbness or tingling in the feet or legs
- slow-healing cuts or bruises
- blurry vision

Know Your Numbers

I hope you will remember one of the key messages of this book—know your numbers. It's a recurring theme because it's such an important step in preventing and managing your risks for heart disease and other health conditions. Whether its diabetes, cholesterol, or blood pressure, knowing your numbers and what they mean are key. As I mentioned, many people do not even know they have diabetes—and in this case, what you don't know can definitely hurt you! So, the first step is to get tested, particularly if you've experienced any of the warning signs for diabetes or you have a family history of the condition.

There are two types of tests used to diagnose diabetes: the fasting glucose test and the hemoglobin A1c (HgA1c) test. The fasting glucose test is the most common and quickest test administered. After you fast for 12 hours, your blood is drawn. Blood sugar can be measured with just one drop of blood from the prick of a finger, which is how those with diabetes test their own blood sugar levels throughout the day. However, a lab will typically draw a vial of blood for complete testing. Results from this test may show blood sugar in the following ranges:

- 65 to 100 mg/dL: indicates a normal blood glucose level
- 101 to 124 mg/dL: indicates an impaired glucose level, or prediabetes
- 125 mg/dL or higher: indicates diabetes

If diabetes is suspected, a patient is often asked to take the HgA1c test. While a fasting glucose test shows your blood sugar at the present moment, the HgA1c measures your blood sugar levels over the past three months by analyzing the hemoglobin. Hemoglobin is the protein molecule in our red blood cells that carries oxygen from the lungs to our body's tissues and returns carbon dioxide to the lungs. When glucose is present in the bloodstream it can attach to these red blood cells; the larger the amount of glucose, the more it sticks to the hemoglobin. Since these blood cells last about three months, they can tell us about blood sugar levels during that time. This more involved analysis is usually necessary to confirm a diagnosis of diabetes.

The American Diabetes Association (ADA) uses the HgA1c to help define prediabetes and diabetes. For instance, a woman who has prediabetes, and is therefore at risk of developing diabetes, will have an elevated HgA1c level—between 5.7 and 6.4 percent. Women with an HgA1c between 6.0 and 6.5 percent have a more than tenfold increased risk of developing diabetes compared to women with lower levels of HgA1c. Results from this test may show HgA1c in the following ranges:
- <5.7 percent—a normal range
- 5.7–6.4 percent—increased risk for prediabetes or diabetes
- 6.5 percent or higher—indicating diabetes

Less than 7.0 percent is the goal for women who currently have diabetes.

Although this test is more involved, some studies suggest that HgA1c is less sensitive than the fasting blood glucose test in detecting prediabetes. With that in mind, I would suggest looking at both numbers, as well as the trend in blood sugar levels over time. Your annual physical examination should include a fasting blood glucose test. If that number is high, or there is a trend toward increased levels, your health-care provider may perform further testing and monitor levels carefully going forward. This is also the time to begin making lifestyle changes to keep blood sugar levels in check.

Knowing your numbers and tracking any trends are important because recognizing prediabetes can help you avoid developing diabetes. By changing your diet and increasing exercise, you can reverse those trends. Your health-care provider may also suggest medications to help you lower your glucose levels, but as with all medications, these drugs will be much more effective when taken in conjunction with lifestyle modifications.

Treatment for Diabetes

Managing diabetes involves regular blood sugar testing, as well as insulin and other medications to control glucose levels. A healthy lifestyle can limit the number and dosage of these medications and can sometimes eliminate the need for them altogether. It's important to work with your health-care provider to find the best medication or combination of medications for you. This often requires a patient to monitor glucose levels closely and then tailoring medications to best fit her individual needs. If you are taking medication for diabetes, be sure to tell your physician about any changes in your activity level or diet.

Of course, having a healthy lifestyle is the best way to prevent diabetes in the first place. It's no surprise that many of the same recommendations for heart health apply to diabetes prevention, as well. This includes a diet high in fruits and vegetables; eating whole grains instead of white flour breads and pasta; avoiding foods that are high in saturated fat, such as fried foods; and

CATHERINE'S STORY

Like many women, Catherine takes her health for granted. At 45, she has no medical problems and has been feeling fine; therefore, she rarely visits her physician. She knows she could be eating better and exercising more, but with a busy family and a full-time job, who has the time?

During the summer, a family reunion was planned. At the big barbecue, a cousin to whom she had been quite close growing up asked her if she was aware of her risk for diabetes. Catherine was surprised and asked why her cousin was concerned. She went on to remind Catherine that several members of her family, including Catherine's mother, had been diagnosed with type 2 diabetes. She also reminded Catherine that during her pregnancy Catherine had experienced problems with elevated blood sugar— gestational diabetes. Since this problem went away after her children were born, Catherine didn't think any more about the matter. Catherine's cousin was worried because she herself had recently been diagnosed with diabetes. She had changed her diet and started to exercise. These lifestyle changes allowed Catherine's cousin to control her blood glucose without medications. However, her diagnosis made her concerned for Catherine's health.

Later that summer, Catherine made an appointment

with her primary care doctor to review her risk for diabetes. The doctor agreed that her lifestyle, coupled with her history of gestational diabetes, placed Catherine at an increased risk for diabetes. In addition, Catherine's increased waist circumference and slightly elevated blood pressure met the criteria for metabolic syndrome. Catherine's doctor told her that having metabolic syndrome increased her risk for diabetes about seven times.

With this newfound information, Catherine started to make walking part of her daily routine. She avoided simple carbohydrates and ate more whole grains, fruits, and vegetables. Without being on a strict diet, Catherine lost about 20 pounds. Her blood pressure improved and was no longer in the high normal or prehypertensive range. Happily, she noticed her waistline had decreased, as well. During a follow-up appointment, her doctor confirmed that these changes had substantially reduced her risk for diabetes. As soon as she arrived home, Catherine called her cousin to give her the good news and thank her for opening her eyes to the risks she had been ignoring. They both agreed that prevention was a powerful weapon and made a date to toast their good health.

limiting desserts and sugar-laden beverages. (See chapters 11 and 12 for a more complete guide to diet and exercise.)

Diabetes Prevention Program

In 2002, the results of a major study were published. This study examined the benefits of diet and exercise in the prevention of diabetes compared to medication. Women (and men) who had prediabetes (everyone had elevated blood glucose levels that were high but not in the diabetes range) were divided into three groups. The first group, which was referred to as the "lifestyle group," received advice on a healthy diet and exercise plan. The second group received no specific advice (just the usual care from their physicians), and the third group was given medication to lower their blood glucose levels. Participants in the lifestyle group were almost 60 percent LESS likely to develop diabetes, compared to the group that did not receive advice on diet and exercise. In fact, the lifestyle group did better than the group who received a medication (metformin) to help prevent diabetes by controlling their blood sugar.

Metabolic Syndrome

There are some factors that place women at higher risk for both diabetes and heart disease. When a woman has three or more of these factors, it is called metabolic syndrome. While metabolic syndrome is recognized around the world, there are slight differences in the criteria used by individual countries to diagnose the condition. In general, the components of metabolic syndrome include excess fat around the waist, elevated blood pressure, high cholesterol, and blood glucose levels in the prediabetes range. In the United States, most physicians use the following criteria to diagnose metabolic syndrome:

- a waist circumference of 35 inches or greater for women
- serum triglycerides* of 150 mg/dL or greater, or use of a

medication to lower triglycerides

- serum HDL cholesterol* of less than 50 mg/dL in women, or use of a medication to raise HDL cholesterol
- fasting blood glucose of 100 mg/dL or more, or use of a medication to lower glucose
- blood pressure of 130/85 mmHg or greater, or use of a medication to lower blood pressure

(*See chapter 7, "The Cholesterol Connection," for more about triglycerides and HDL cholesterol levels.)

Having three or more of these factors means you have met the criteria for metabolic syndrome and are at an increased risk for diabetes, heart disease, and stroke. A special note should be made regarding waist circumference for women who are Asian (South Asian, Chinese, or Japanese, etc.). For these women, the risk of diabetes occurs at lower waist circumference levels (31.5 inches). The bottom line is that increased belly fat is a cause for concern. This type of fat will significantly increase your risk of diabetes and heart disease. Ask your physician or health-care professional to review the criteria for metabolic syndrome with you. Again, knowing your numbers is important. If you know your waist circumference and begin to see it growing, you can take steps to get back on track.

Gestational Diabetes

Women have a special concern about diabetes during pregnancy. When a woman has high blood glucose levels during pregnancy, we call this gestational diabetes. Women with a history of gestational diabetes are at an increased risk for developing diabetes (and thus heart disease) later in life; therefore, understanding this type of diabetes is an important component of heart health. Between 2 and 10 percent of women will develop gestational diabetes while pregnant.

This is worrisome because gestational diabetes increases a woman's risk for complications both before and after birth. For instance, the condition increases the chances of a woman giving birth to a large baby, which may make labor and delivery difficult. Gestational diabetes also increases the risk for developing pre-eclampsia, a serious condition marked by dangerously high blood pressure, and can be life threatening for both mother and child.

Gestational Diabetes Risk Factors

- age over 25 years when pregnant
- a family history of diabetes
- having high blood pressure prior to pregnancy
- being overweight before pregnancy
- a prior pregnancy during which you had gestational diabetes

Symptoms of gestational diabetes may include:

- blurred vision
- extreme fatigue
- increased urination and thirst
- sudden changes in weight, such as weight loss

Some women may also be more susceptible to infections or feel continually nauseous. If you are pregnant and experience any of these warning signs, you should have your blood sugar tested right away. The earlier you recognize the problem, the sooner you can prevent complications for you and your baby.

It's common for an obstetrician to monitor blood glucose levels during pregnancy, but be sure to let your health-care provider know about any risk factors you may have for gestational diabetes. Generally, an obstetrician or midwife will screen for gestational diabetes between 24 and 28 weeks into the pregnancy, but this testing may occur earlier if you have risk factors. The test is simple: you are asked to drink a sugary (glucose) beverage, and then your blood is drawn and checked for elevated levels of glucose. If your glucose level is high after a certain period of time, it means you are not producing enough insulin to regulate your blood sugar.

Treatment for Gestational Diabetes

If you do develop gestational diabetes, your health-care provider can help you manage your blood glucose levels during pregnancy. Sometimes that means taking medications, but lifestyle changes are always an important part of managing this condition. Just like regular diabetes, gestational diabetes can be prevented and controlled with a healthy diet that:

- is high in fruits and vegetables;
- includes whole-grain carbohydrates (as opposed to refined or white flour);
- avoids high-calorie, sugary foods such as soda and other sweetened beverages, candy, or desserts; and avoids high-fat foods, and includes healthy saturated fats such as olive or canola oil

With the guidance of your health-care provider, you should also include exercise daily. Even a 20-minute walk can help control blood sugar, lower blood pressure, and keep your weight under control. Your heart will also thank you!

With gestational diabetes, it's important to monitor both mother and baby closely during the pregnancy, throughout labor and delivery, and into the postpartum period. Therefore, make sure to keep all your doctor's appointments, which may be more frequent. The good news is, most women will have lower blood sugar levels after delivery, and diabetes medications such as insulin can often be discontinued. However, you should never stop taking medications without the advice of your physician.

After Delivery: Future Risk for Diabetes

An estimated 33 to 66 percent of women with gestational diabetes will develop the condition again with future pregnancies. The chances also increase with age—women who have gestational diabetes during pregnancy have a much higher risk (about eight times higher) of diabetes as they get older. In addition, women who have gestational diabetes and are overweight significantly increase their chances of developing type 2 diabetes after pregnancy. Between 50 and 75 percent of women who have gestational diabetes and are overweight (i.e., obese) will develop type 2 diabetes. As mentioned before, excess fat around the waistline is the most common risk factor. Even women who are considered normal weight have a slightly increased risk for developing diabetes in the future once they've had gestational diabetes—about 25 percent or less. But again, type 2 diabetes can be prevented with dietary changes, regular exercise, and weight loss.

Considering this increased risk, it's important for women who have had gestational diabetes to have their blood glucose monitored regularly throughout their lifetimes. The possibility of developing type 2 diabetes becomes greater with time—from a 5 percent increase in the first year after pregnancy to a 20 percent increase ten years down the road. Therefore, the American Diabetes Association recommends:

- Annual glucose monitoring for women age 45 or greater at the time of pregnancy with gestational diabetes
- Testing every three years for women under the age of 45 years with gestational diabetes

Why is this so important for heart health? A woman with a history of gestational diabetes is at an increased risk for developing heart disease. Even if your blood glucose levels were close to normal and you did not need medication to keep it under control during your pregnancy, having gestational diabetes still puts you at greater risk for developing diabetes and heart disease at an earlier age, compared to women with normal glucose levels throughout their pregnancies.

Take a Step

To sum things up, what's good for diabetes prevention and management is also good for your heart. That's great news for all us multitasking women! Leading a healthy lifestyle can significantly reduce your chances of developing diabetes, as well as heart disease. In addition to following recommended dietary and exercise guidelines, here are a few simple steps you can take to ward off diabetes:

- Get Tested—Find out what your fasting glucose level is and keep track of any changes. If you have risk factors, such as a family history of diabetes, you may need to be tested more often. Also, if your fasting blood glucose level has been elevated in the past (over 100 mg/dL) then more frequent monitoring is recommended. Remember, a diagnosis of prediabetes gives you an opportunity to reduce your blood sugar with lifestyle changes and prevent type 2 diabetes.
- Get Treated—Sometimes, despite lifestyle changes, blood sugar levels remain high. For certain women with prediabetes or metabolic syndrome, medications together with diet and exercise are the best management. Talk to your health-care provider about what's right for you.

CHAPTER NINE

Smoke-Free for Life

What comes from the heart, goes to the heart.

SAMUEL COLERIDGE

It's no secret that smoking is bad for your health. By now, you've probably heard the warnings regarding emphysema, bronchitis, and lung cancer. However, the health risks associated with cigarette smoking and tobacco use go far beyond those diseases. Because smoking causes cellular damage, it also increases your risk of developing nearly all forms of cancer. In fact, smoking harms every organ in your body, including your heart. And, here's something else that may surprise you: while both men and women who smoke are at a dramatically increased risk for heart disease and stroke, evidence suggests that a woman's risk from smoking may be greater than a man's. Studies have shown that **among men and women age 35 to 52 years, the number of heart attacks is six times greater for women smokers compared to women who do not smoke,** while the risk for men who smoke is three times greater than for nonsmoking men. In a large study done in Copenhagen, women who smoked were found to have a nine times greater risk of heart attack versus the three times increased risk observed in men! What's more alarming is that many of the women in these studies reported smoking just a few cigarettes per day or only smoking "socially," which means that even occasional or moderate smoking significantly increases your risk for heart attack. When it comes to smoking, there is no "safe" amount.

How Smoking Affects the Heart

Although the warnings we hear about smoking tend to focus on the respiratory system, more smokers actually die from heart attacks. In fact, for men and women under age 50, cigarette smoking is the most important risk factor for cardiovascular disease. Smokers also experience cardiac events, such as heart attacks, about 13 years earlier than nonsmokers. That means that young women who smoke have a very real chance of suffering a heart attack. Not only do smokers increase their risk of developing cardiovascular disease, women who smoke tend to have more complications after a heart attack when compared to men. In other words, the threats posed by cigarettes are serious. Smoking causes damage to the circulatory system and the heart in a number of ways:

The adverse effects from cigarette smoking account for an estimated 443,000 deaths (or one out of every five deaths) each year in the United States—that's more than all deaths from HIV, illegal drug use, alcohol use, car accidents, suicides, and murders combined. However, smoking is also the most *preventable* cause of disease and death. Within minutes of your last cigarette, your health begins to improve.

- Once inhaled, harmful substances in cigarettes enter the bloodstream and damage the walls of your arteries. In the same way that injury from high blood pressure, high cholesterol, and diabetes makes the arteries more susceptible to atherosclerosis, smoking leads to plaque formation and heart disease.

- As arteries become narrower, circulation decreases while your blood pressure and heart rate increase, putting more strain on the cardiovascular system. In addition, blood vessels get stiffer when exposed to the toxins in cigarette smoke, which increases your blood pressure and thins blood vessels, making them more likely to form plaque.

- Smoking reduces oxygen levels in the blood, so your organs (including your heart) do not receive the oxygen they need to function properly. Over time, this decrease in oxygen can permanently damage organs and impair the body's ability to heal.

- Smoking also increases your chances of forming a blood clot, which can lead to a heart attack or stroke. Smokers have high levels of inflammation in their bodies, which we now know leads to plaque instability. Unstable plaque, if you recall, is more likely to break open (rupture) and cause a clot. Remember, these types of clots are the central component of heart attacks and ischemic strokes.

- Finally, smoking contributes to unhealthy cholesterol. It both decreases HDL (good) cholesterol and worsens the effects of LDL (bad) cholesterol. There is some evidence to suggest that women who smoke reduce their HDL levels to a greater degree than men who smoke.

Why does smoking affect women's risk for heart events so dramatically? Although some of the exact cause and effect is still a mystery, it's believed that smoking may reduce estrogen levels. If you remember, estrogen does offer premenopausal women some protection against heart disease; so if estrogen levels are decreased, this protection also disappears. In addition, women have smaller arteries than men, which makes plaque buildup more serious. While we continue to research the effects of smoking on the cardiovascular system, we do know this: if you don't smoke, you reduce your risk of heart disease.

Stroke Risks

Smoking also increases a woman's risk for stroke. An estimated 25 percent of all strokes are related to the effects of smoking. Among women enrolled in the Nurses' Health Study, the risk for stroke in women who smoked was almost three times that of non-smokers. The reasons for this increased risk are the same as we listed earlier for heart disease: smoking damages blood vessels, leads to atherosclerosis, and raises the chances of forming a blood clot, which can cause a blocked artery to the brain or stroke. Again, according to the American Heart Association, women who smoke have a much higher risk of developing dangerous blood clots, ischemic strokes, and certain types of brain hemorrhage, as compared to men who smoke. The risks for coronary artery disease and stroke become even greater for women who smoke *and* use oral contraceptives or hormone replacement therapy.

Secondhand Smoke

If you don't quit smoking for yourself, you may consider quitting for those around you. Nonsmokers exposed to secondhand smoke are at a 25 percent higher risk of developing heart disease than nonsmokers who are not exposed to cigarette smoke. According to the Centers for Disease Control and Prevention, an estimated 46,000 premature deaths from heart disease each year are due to the effects of secondhand smoke. This means that even if you don't

> Did you know that secondhand smoke contains 7,000 chemicals—hundreds of which are toxic—and 70 that are known to cause cancer? There is no "risk-free" level of secondhand smoke.

smoke, but are exposed to secondhand smoke at home or work, your risk of heart disease and stroke is increased. Even brief exposure can damage the lining of your blood vessels and cause your blood platelets to become "stickier." Therefore, people who already have heart disease or have experienced a heart attack are at an especially high risk and should avoid any exposure to secondhand smoke.

Fortunately, the number of people who report their homes as "smoke free" has climbed in recent years. In addition, many local and statewide policies now prohibit smoking in public places, which greatly reduces our exposure to secondhand smoke. Still, there is work to be done. Studies show that 40 to 56 percent of nonsmokers have detectable levels of cotinine, a chemical found in cigarettes, in their blood, which indicates exposure to secondhand smoke. If we continue to reduce secondhand smoke, we will likely see reductions in rates of heart disease. Whether you are trying to quit the habit, or supporting a family member or friend in his or her efforts to stop smoking, you are making a valuable contribution to the prevention of heart disease for yourself and those around you.

Smoking Trends

To me, one of the most worrying statistics regarding smoking is that, despite the overwhelming evidence, a large number of teens and young adults continue to smoke. In a recent study, over 45 percent of high school students reported smoking at least one cigarette, and 19.5 percent admitted to smoking regularly. Even more disturbing is that among women ages 15 to 44 years, the rate of smoking is estimated at 27.4 percent, which is higher than the national average of 19.3 percent for all adults 18 years or older. Rates are highest among non-Hispanic white women and non-Hispanic black women, as well as Native American and Native Alaskan women. When you consider that women who smoke, on average, die almost 15 years earlier than nonsmoking women, these statistics are even more sobering.

> The costs of smoking are staggering. Medical costs related to smoking are estimated at $96 billion annually, while losses in worker productivity related to smoking are estimated at $193 billion per year!

Since most adult smokers start the habit when they are preteens or teenagers, I believe it's very important to educate children and teens, particularly young women, on the dangers of smoking from an early age and continuing into adulthood. Remind your teens that there is nothing "cool" about cancer or heart disease! Parents can also serve as positive role models by choosing not to smoke, or quitting. Online resources such as www.kidshealth.org can help parents start a dialogue and provide teens with information in a language they understand.

Kick the Habit—Improve Your Health!

The good news is the health benefits of being smoke free are immediate and get better over time. The body is truly amazing in its ability to heal. For instance, nicotine stops constricting your blood vessels within 20 minutes of your last cigarette. Your heart rate slows down and your blood pressure decreases. Even your circulation begins to improve. After eight to ten hours without a cigarette, carbon monoxide levels in your bloodstream drop, while oxygen levels increase. Within 24 hours, your risk of having a heart attack is already reduced. And things just keep improving. Studies show that after a smoke-free year, the risks to your health are cut in half, and your body continues to mend with each passing year.

If reducing your risk for cancer and heart disease, along with a host of other ailments is not enough, consider these additional benefits of kicking the habit:

- You'll be helping others, especially the people closest to you, avoid developing serious health problems. Secondhand smoke not only increases the risk of heart disease in adults, it causes asthma attacks, respiratory infections, and ear infections in infants and children, and has been linked to sudden infant death syndrome (SIDS).
- You'll save money. If you add up the savings from not buying cigarettes, plus the money you can avoid spending on medical bills, it can be significant. Think of the things you could do with that extra cash!

How to Quit

Nicotine is as addictive as heroin, so quitting is not easy. In fact, some of my patients have told me that throwing away their cigarettes is the one of the hardest things they've ever done—but also the most rewarding. In addition to potentially adding years to your life, people who stop smoking are often pleasantly surprised by other perks. Many folks find their sense of smell and taste improves dramatically. They also tend to get fewer colds, coughs, and sinus problems. And, since they are able to breathe more easily, nonsmokers usually have more energy. In addition, many women find their complexions look better. Since smoking does cause wrinkles, quitting may be one of the best anti-aging secrets out there! But, of course, first you have to quit.

Fortunately, there is a wealth of information and numerous smoking cessation products available to help you kick the habit. Web sites such as www.smokefree.gov and The American Lung Association's www.lung.org/stop-smoking provide advice, support, and step-by-step guidelines. Tech savvy women can find free mobile apps such as QuitGuide to help you stay on track.

However, the most valuable resource is your health-care provider. He or she can recommend over-the-counter products or prescribe medications to help you avoid withdrawal symptoms and give you the willpower you need to get through a very difficult process. Some of those options include:

- **Nicotine gum, lozenges, and patches**—By providing a low level of nicotine, without the other toxins present during smoking, these products can help you manage withdrawal symptoms. Be sure to follow the directions on the package very carefully. Though these aids are available over the counter, it's advisable to work with your physician when you decide to quit smoking. Quitting may affect other medications you are on, and some nicotine replacement products can cause health problems if not used properly.

- **Nicotine inhalers and nasal sprays**—Both of these medications require a prescription, but have proven to be highly effective. Inhalers and sprays deliver nicotine into your body in a similar fashion as smoking, and because it's absorbed quickly, it provides immediate relief for a nicotine craving.

- **Bupropion**—This oral medication, which is also known as Wellbutrin or Zyban, is available only by prescription. Unlike nicotine replacement products, bupropion reduces cravings and withdrawal symptoms by altering certain chemicals in the brain. It was originally developed as an antidepressant, but was found to be very effective as a smoking cessation aid for some people. Like any medication, bupropion does come with a risk for side effects and may not be right for everyone.

I would like to add a special caution regarding nicotine poisoning. It's very important to not smoke while using one of the nicotine replacement products listed above. These aids provide your body with nicotine, which is a poison, and too much will cause an overdose. Symptoms of nicotine poisoning may include weakness, dizziness, severe headaches, nausea, vomiting, diarrhea, cold sweats, blurred vision, hearing difficulties, or mental confusion. If you suspect nicotine poisoning, call your physician or go to an emergency room right away.

As noted, quitting the cigarette habit and staying smoke free can be extremely challenging. Many people try to quit smoking multiple times before they are successful. You should not be discouraged and give up if you relapse; simply try again. Keep in mind, social support has been found to be the most important factor in whether you succeed. So, be sure to enlist the help of family and friends when you decide to quit. You may also consider joining a support group, either in person or online. The American Cancer Society, the American Heart Association, and the American Lung Association can point you in the right direction.

Choosing not to smoke is one of the best ways to prevent heart disease. We hope we made the dangers of smoking very clear, and perhaps provided the nudge you need to quit. Your heart, along with the rest of your body, will thank you. As mentioned, there are many online resources, as well as information from your health-care provider that can assist you in the process of quitting. However, if you are thinking about kicking the habit (and we hope you are!), here are few tips to get you started:

1. Pick a date to quit and mark it on your calendar.

2. Tell family and friends your quit date and enlist their support.

3. Write the three most important reasons why you want to quit on a card (e.g., *I want to be healthy and energetic enough to play with my grandchildren, I want to set a good example for my teenage daughter, I want to travel when I retire*, etc.), post the card in a visible place and look at it several times a day.

4. Talk to your health-care provider about nicotine replacement therapies and get a prescription if necessary.

5. Stock up on cigarette "replacements," such sugarless gum, sugarless hard candy, and healthy snacks. Be sure to carry a supply with you in your purse and/or car.

6. Consider joining a smoking cessation class or support group.

7. Get rid of all cigarettes, ashtrays, lighters, and matches.

8. Remember the four "As" to handle cravings:
   a. AVOID people and places that tempt you to smoke.
   b. ALTER some of your daily habits, such as your route to work or mealtimes
   c. ALTERNATIVES for your mouth—sugarless gum and candy, healthy snacks
   d. ACTIVITIES for your hands—start a hobby such as knitting

9. Join an exercise class or walk regularly with a friend to stay active.

10. Make a follow-up appointment with your physician to track your progress.

CHAPTER TEN

A Change of Heart

It's not enough to change your mind; the most lasting and meaningful transformations require a change of heart.

UNKNOWN

One of the most important factors influencing our risk for heart disease is lifestyle. If we all lived a healthy lifestyle—eating fresh, wholesome foods, getting regular exercise, not smoking, and reducing stress—about 75 percent of all heart attacks could be prevented. In other words, most people can avoid heart disease, as well as high cholesterol, hypertension, and diabetes, by simply changing their behaviors. Even if you have a family history of heart disease, you can dramatically reduce your risk by adopting healthy habits (genes account for only so much). In addition to dodging heart attacks and strokes, good lifestyle choices can help you enjoy a better quality of life.

Information is only part of the equation. Learning about risk factors and how to improve your health is only beneficial if you put that knowledge into practice. The evidence regarding the benefits of a healthy lifestyle is undeniable, and surveys suggest that many people believe they should make better choices (i.e., stop smoking, improve their diets, exercise more often). Yet, health problems like heart disease and diabetes are still on the rise, which begs the question: why aren't more people making positive lifestyle changes?

First of all, change can be hard. Those of us who have reached middle age or older have spent a lifetime developing eating habits and attitudes toward exercise that may be difficult to modify—difficult, but not impossible! Secondly, our modern culture contributes to our unhealthy lifestyles and often makes it more challenging to embrace the changes we know we should make.

A Recipe for Poor Health

Harmful Eating Habits We are busy people. Between careers, family obligations, household chores, errands, and hopefully squeezing in a few hours for ourselves, we have very little time and energy left over. Because of this time crunch, we often reach for the most convenient foods—premade or packaged meals, Chinese takeout, pizza delivery, and other fast food options. (As a working mom, I have been known to order pizza in a pinch!) These foods may be convenient, but they are typically high in calories and loaded with harmful fat, sugar, and sodium. What's worse, over time, we develop a taste for these foods and find ourselves craving more and more. These poor eating habits have contributed to an increase in obesity, hypertension, diabetes, high cholesterol, and, of course, cardiovascular problems.

It takes more time and energy to prepare natural, whole foods, but the benefits are certainly worth the effort. Not only can a healthy diet prevent many diseases, studies show that eating well can be more effective than prescription medications at reducing cholesterol, lowering blood pressure, and controlling blood sugar.

We will talk more about what constitutes a healthy diet, as well as tips to make it easier, in the next chapter, "Eating for Life." For now, suffice it to say that a diet consisting primarily of whole grains, fruits and vegetables, and low-fat and minimally processed foods is essential for good health.

Lack of Exercise Another by-product of our culture is the lack of physical activity. Thanks to many modern conveniences, we have become very sedentary beings. We no longer have to hunt and gather, or tend to fields in order to put food on the table. We travel in cars, buses, or subways instead of walking. We use elevators instead of stairs. Many of us perform our jobs while sitting in front of a computer all day. Even much of our entertainment (television and video games) requires no movement. Again, this makes life more convenient, but it wreaks havoc on our health.

The human body was designed for activity. Regular exercise is necessary to keep our bodies functioning properly and maintain strong, flexible muscles—including our hearts. Many health problems, such as high blood pressure, high cholesterol, diabetes, obesity, and heart disease, can be prevented or controlled by adding more activity to our daily routines. In chapter 12, we'll discuss further the role exercise plays in our health, as well as ways to stay active.

Excessive Stress Modern living can also produce undue stress. You can argue that stress is nothing new—humans have always dealt with it. Stress is actually a natural physiological response (sometimes referred to as the "fight or flight" response) that can help us survive a life-threatening situation. However, instead of the stress we might experience if we were being chased by a bear, for instance, the anxiety we experience today tends to be chronic mental and emotional stress. When stress levels remain consistently high, hormones such as adrenaline and cortisol raise blood sugar and constrict blood vessels, which then increases blood pressure. Unmanaged stress can also increase your LDL (bad) cholesterol and triglycerides, while decreasing your HDL (good) cholesterol. We will delve deeper into how stress contributes to heart disease, as well as how you can manage it more effectively, in chapter 13.

As you can see, the combination of harmful eating habits, lack of exercise, and chronic stress, all common in today's world, is a potent recipe for poor health.

Nurses' Health Study

One of the studies I like to review with medical students and doctors in training is the Nurses' Health Study, which is the largest and longest running study of women's health issues. Researchers at Harvard took data from this study and examined dietary patterns together with other lifestyle behaviors. What they found makes sense. Women who did not smoke, were active (exercising 30 minutes per day), were at a healthy weight, and ate a healthy diet were much less likely to have a heart attack or stroke, or become diabetic. In fact, women who optimized these behaviors were about 80 to 90 percent less likely to have one or more of these outcomes (heart attack, stroke, or diabetes).

To learn more about the Nurses' Health Study, visit www.nhs3.org.

Making Changes

If you've ever made and broken a New Year's resolution, you know how difficult changing behaviors can be. You're not alone. In fact, researchers in behavioral medicine have spent a great deal of time studying the process of change. As you might expect, people tend to approach change in very different ways. Some folks are very adaptable and like to dive right in, while others would rather test the waters of change slowly. Additionally, change is often a process of trial and error, requiring many attempts before any meaningful transformations occur. The important thing is to keep trying!

In general, the process of change can be separated into five stages—pre-contemplation, contemplation, preparation, action, and maintenance. By understanding these stages, you may gain some insight into what is holding you back from making positive lifestyle changes and help you succeed. Let's take a quick look at each step in the process.

Pre-Contemplation In this stage, a person is not ready for change. He or she is not modifying any behaviors and doesn't intend to make changes. The person may not have the necessary tools or information to take a positive step forward, or may feel a lack of control over the situation. Denial is also common in this stage (e.g., "Smoking is not really bad for my health"). Unfortunately, someone in this stage may consider it easier to stay in a particular situation, even if it means living with health problems and a shortened life expectancy, than to make a change for the better. To move someone past this stage, you can explain the risks associated with current habits and encourage them to rethink their behaviors.

Contemplation Since you're reading this book, there's a good chance you are in the contemplation stage or beyond. A person in this stage knows it's better to live a healthier lifestyle, but hasn't taken any action yet. This is a time for gathering information, weighing the pros and cons, and perhaps talking to a health-care provider about what steps to take. Many people in this stage feel conflicted about giving something up, but the focus should not be on what you give up, but rather on what you gain. If you are contemplating change, learning about your risk factors along with the benefits of a healthy lifestyle is an important first step.

Preparation Maybe you've dug your walking shoes out from the back of the closet or purchased a book of heart-healthy recipes. If so, you're probably in the preparation stage. This is where you begin to take small steps toward a healthier lifestyle. In this stage, it's important to stay motivated. Try writing down your goals or preparing a plan of action. Other strategies may include posting inspirational quotes on the fridge or putting reminders in your calendar, keeping your workout clothes/shoes easily accessible, or signing up for an exercise class with a friend. The advice and support of family and friends can be very helpful at this stage.

Action During this stage, you begin to take direct action toward achieving your goal, such as starting a regular exercise routine and/or adopting healthy eating habits. Studies show that it takes about two months to develop a new habit, and that as many as 50 percent of people who start a new routine drop out in the first six months. Therefore, it's important to stick with your changes during those first challenging months by rewarding your successes, seeking the support of family and friends, and posting reminders of your ultimate goal. Think about how quickly two months fly by! Before you know it, you will have established a new healthy habit.

Maintenance Once you've maintained a regular exercise program or followed a heart-healthy diet for at least six months, you've reached the maintenance stage. Here's the good news—healthy habits can become second nature. Many people find they have gotten so used to their new habits that missing a morning walk or a regular workout is very disappointing. The new activity becomes an enjoyable part of their daily routine. After six months of eating well, people often lose their taste for processed food. This is also the stage during which the benefits of a healthy lifestyle become more apparent (e.g., lower blood pressure, reduced cholesterol, weight loss, or increased energy) providing motivation to continue. Even so, it's vital to develop coping strategies to deal with temptation in this stage.

If you reach the maintenance phase, congratulate yourself, but don't let your guard down! Relapse is common, so it's important to stay motivated. You might consider adding some fun activities into your regular exercise routine, trying a new sport, or experimenting with some fresh heart-healthy recipes. If you relapse, don't be too hard on yourself, and don't give up. Try to identify the reasons why you fell back into an old routine, and ask yourself how you can avoid these triggers in the future. Then take another stride forward. Every step you take toward a healthier lifestyle reduces your risk for heart disease.

A recent campaign by the American Heart Association, which promotes awareness of heart disease, puts it best: "If you are doing nothing, do something. If you are doing something, do a little more."

Take a Step

Changing your lifestyle can seem overwhelming. I often counsel my patients to change one thing at a time—say, reducing saturated fat or sodium in their diets or walking for 20 minutes each day. Once you've successfully changed one habit, you can focus on another. Each step you take toward heart health becomes easier and more effective. To get started on the road to change, you can:

- **Spend a few minutes thinking about why you want to make a change.** What is your true motivation? Your physician may have said you need to lower your blood pressure, but the reason for controlling your blood pressure is not to satisfy your doctor; it's to improve your health and prolong your life. Therefore, being healthy enough to travel when you retire or having the energy to play with your grandchildren may be your true motivation. It's also important to focus on the immediate feelings of healthy actions, which will keep you motivated day to day.

- **Write down your goals.** It's helpful to commit your goals to paper and create a plan of action, and then post it in a visible location. Be specific! The more specific your goals, the more likely you are to succeed. For instance, "I will walk for 30 minutes every day" is more achievable and effective than "I will increase my activity level." By the same token, obtaining and following a heart-healthy diet will produce better results than simply saying "I will eat better."

- **Don't be afraid to ask for help.** Your health-care provider can be a valuable resource. He or she can provide free dietary and exercise guidelines to follow. In addition, there are many online resources available (see the Resources section in the back of the book). If you are feeling overwhelmed, you might consider consulting a nutritionist or personal trainer, who can help get you on track and keep you motivated. Enlisting the support of family or friends can also be helpful.

- **Treat yourself.** Sometimes the best motivation is a reward. Tell yourself you'll schedule a massage or plan a weekend getaway with the girls if you stick to your exercise routine for two months. Buy a new pair of walking shoes or invest in a great heart-healthy cookbook, if that's what it takes to get you started.

- **Learn more.** Read the following chapters on diet, exercise, and stress reduction so you know what it takes to be heart healthy for life!

CHAPTER ELEVEN

Eating for Life

The most indispensable ingredient of all good home cooking: love, for those you are cooking for. It should come from the heart.

SOPHIA LOREN

Diet is a central component of a healthy lifestyle. The connection between food and your health is very powerful; a good diet can ward off high blood pressure, diabetes, elevated cholesterol, and obesity. With the exception of smoking, that's all the major risk factors for heart disease! In fact, studies show that poor eating patterns are a major contributor to heart disease.

Unfortunately, for the majority of us, diet is one of the most difficult things to change. Not only are eating habits often firmly entrenched since childhood, certain foods can evoke feelings of comfort, which make them hard to give up. There can also be a great deal of confusion about what constitutes a healthy diet. It seems as though every week a new study is published outlining what's good for us and what's not. No wonder many of my patients come into the office feeling frustrated about what to eat!

Ironically, for centuries our ancestors, who had very little information or choice regarding the food they ate, were able to eat a far healthier diet, without thinking much about it. Today, the availability and variety of foods we have make eating more interesting and convenient, but often less healthy. That's because the foods that are most plentiful and easiest to consume are typically highly processed and loaded with fat, sugar, and sodium, but low in nutrients. It may take a little more time and effort to feed yourself and your family a healthy diet, but the rewards are definitely worth it.

It's true: "You are what you eat." Your body uses nutrients from the food you eat for cellular growth and repair, as well as fuel for energy. Numerous studies show that a healthy diet can lower blood pressure, reduce cholesterol, and prevent diabetes, therefore reducing your risk for cardiovascular disease. What's more, a good diet can be more powerful than medications—with fewer adverse side effects. In fact, the "side effects" of a healthy diet may include weight loss, increased energy, better quality of life, and more years to enjoy it!

Eating well may require some effort, but it doesn't have to be complicated. In this chapter, we will focus on the key aspects of a healthy diet, along with ways we can improve our food choices and maintain these changes—and that's the important part. No diet is beneficial unless you stick with it. That's why fad diets and eating plans that severely limit your choices don't work over the long term. While I use the word "diet," I don't want you to think of a short-term, restrictive plan, but rather developing good eating habits for life.

Heart-Healthy Diet Basics

When it comes to preventing heart disease and stroke, most experts agree on the following dietary guidelines regarding fats, cholesterol, protein, carbohydrates (fiber), fruits and vegetables, and sodium.

Not All Fats Are Created Equal

We need some fat in our diet. Fat supplies energy and provides essential fatty acids for growth, healthy skin, and metabolism. It also helps our bodies absorb certain vitamins. And, let's face it, fat adds flavor, and, because it makes us feel fuller, it can stave off hunger. However, not all fats are the same: some fats are healthy and some are harmful. Saturated fats and trans fats, in particular, are unhealthy and should be limited in your diet.

Saturated Fats In general, saturated fats are solid fats (i.e., they are solid at room temperature)—think of a stick of butter. Saturated fats are mainly derived from animal products such as meat, dairy, and eggs, but can also be found in some plant-based products including coconut, palm, and palm kernel oils.

What makes saturated fats so bad for the body is that they directly raise total and LDL (bad) cholesterol levels. Because of this, the American Heart Association recommends that you consume 7 percent or less of your total calories from saturated fats. To cut down on saturated fats, you should:

- Choose lean meats—Limit red meat (especially red meat that is visibly marbled with fat) and look for cuts labeled "lean" or "extra lean." Poultry (without the skin), veal, lamb, and fish are better choices.
- Trim excess fat from meats before cooking.
- Substitute lean ground turkey or chicken for beef and pork.
- Remove the skin from poultry before cooking, and avoid buying chicken cooked with the skin on.
- Broil, grill, roast, or bake meats on racks that allow fats to drain off.
- Limit or avoid processed meats, such as lunch meat, salami, bologna, pepperoni, or sausage.

- Serve smaller portions of meat and bigger portions of vegetables and whole grains. A serving size of meat is 3 to 4 ounces, which is about the size of a deck of cards.
- Buy low-fat or nonfat dairy products, such as skim milk, low-fat cottage cheese, and nonfat yogurt.
- Limit the use of butter, and if you do use it, spread it sparingly.
- Save high-fat hard or creamy cheeses for special occasions, and keep portions small.
- Use canola, sunflower, vegetable, or olive oils when cooking.

To further assist you, there are many online references and food diaries that make it easy to determine the percentage of saturated fats in a variety of foods.

Trans Fats Trans fats are even more harmful to the body than saturated fats. Not only do they increase total and LDL (bad) cholesterol levels, trans fats decrease HDL (good) cholesterol. Therefore, no amount of trans fat is considered healthy.

Though small quantities of trans fats are found naturally in some dairy and meat products, most trans fats are created artificially. Because trans fats do not "go bad" as quickly as other types of fats, they are used to extend the shelf life of processed foods, such as margarine, cereals, chips, crackers, and bakery goods (e.g., cookies, cakes, and donuts). Many fried foods also contain trans fat, which is soaked up during the cooking process. Until recently, trans fats were widely used in commercial cooking and packaged foods. Now that we know how they contribute to heart disease, strokes, and even diabetes, public health policies have required manufacturers to clearly label the amount of trans fat in their products, and many manufacturers have reduced or eliminated them. Today, even many fast food chains provide nutritional information, including the amount of fats, in the foods they offer.

You have probably seen packaging that reads "no trans fat." Actually, that label may be a bit misleading, since any food that has less than 0.50 grams of trans fat can still make that claim. Instead of relying on the advertising, your best bet is to carefully read the ingredient list and nutritional information. Any product that contains *hydrogenated oil* or *partially hydrogenated oil* also contains trans fat. To reduce the amount of trans fat in your diet:

- Avoid buying commercially prepared baked goods, snack foods, and processed foods, as well as many fast foods. If you do buy these products, read labels carefully.
- Avoid deep fried foods whenever possible.
- Use liquid vegetable oils or cooking sprays that contain no trans fat, instead of shortening, lard, margarine, or butter.
- Avoid margarine containing hydrogenated oils.

If you live with teenagers, as I do, avoiding French fries and other fast foods can be a challenge. Educating children on the effects of these foods from an early age can help, as well as setting a good example by not eating them yourself. I also approach nutrition from a sports standpoint. My boys will listen better if they think nutrition can give them an edge in a sport! In fact, many sports professionals work very hard on their diets, so this can reinforce the message at home.

Monounsaturated and Polyunsaturated Fats The good guys of the fat world are monounsaturated and polyunsaturated fats. As you can probably guess, these fats or oils are liquid at room temperature. Unsaturated fats have the ability to lower LDL (bad) cholesterol and increase HDL (good) cholesterol. In fact, replacing saturated fats with unsaturated fats has been shown to reduce the risk for heart disease.

In addition to improving your cholesterol profile, monounsaturated fats are high in vitamin E, which is an excellent antioxidant.

Good examples of monounsaturated fats are many of the cooking oils we now use, including olive, canola, sunflower, sesame, and peanut oils. Foods such as avocados and nuts (almonds, cashews, or peanuts) are also high in monounsaturated fats.

Polyunsaturated fats are found in plants and vegetables (e.g., soybean, sesame, corn, and cottonseed oils), as well as oil from deep-water fatty fish. Walnuts also contain polyunsaturated fats. In addition, polyunsaturated fats provide essential fatty acids known as omega 6 and omega 3. Most of the plant-based polyunsaturated fats fall into the omega-6 category, while those from fish are generally from the omega-3 group.

Omega-3 Fatty Acids The omega-3 fatty acids found in fish oil have been shown to lessen death from heart disease, as well as reduce stroke, particularly among men and women who have a history of heart disease. Omega-3 has also been shown to prevent sudden death due to abnormal heart rhythms. For this reason, the American Heart Association recommends eating fish at least two times per week. To reap the benefits of omega-3, choose fatty fish, such as salmon, herring, trout, sardines, mackerel, and albacore tuna. Data from several studies, when combined, suggest that consuming fish high in omega-3, even once a week, can reduce your risk for heart disease by about 15 percent.

However, some people should use caution when eating fish. Children and pregnant women have been advised by the U.S. Food and Drug Administration not to eat fish that have the potential for high levels of mercury—this includes swordfish, tilefish, and shark. For the rest of us, the benefits of eating fish generally outweigh the concerns over mercury. Even seafood that typically has low levels of mercury, such as shellfish, canned light tuna, salmon, and catfish, is safe for general consumption and provide heart-healthy omega-3 acids. Like all the food you purchase, you should know as much as possible about the source of your fish. Reputable grocers and fish markets will provide information on where the fish comes from, as well as the potential for mercury.

For those people who don't like to eat fish, I recommend getting omega-3 fatty acids from plant sources. Soybeans, flaxseed, canola oil, and walnuts are all good choices. These foods contain alpha-linolenic acid, which is an omega-3 fatty acid. One note: if you choose to include flaxseed in your diet, it must be ground up in order for the body to absorb the oils properly, and cooking it will destroy the beneficial oils. Ground flaxseed can be sprinkled on foods such as cereal and yogurt. Flaxseed oil can be used in salad dressings or on pasta, but should not be used to cook.

What about omega-3 supplements? First, you should always check with your physician before taking any supplements, particularly if you are taking medications such as blood thinners. If there are no potential interactions, you can take fish oil supplements to get a healthy dose of omega 3. In general, about 1–2 grams per day is a good amount for patients with a history of heart disease. For individuals with high triglycerides, higher doses are sometimes recommended—about 3–4 grams per day. Again, I would suggest buying your supplements from a reputable source to ensure you are getting oils that are filtered and pure.

The bottom line on fats: Even "healthy" fats should be consumed in moderation. Current guidelines suggest the number of calories from fats should be about 25 to 35 percent or less of your total daily calories. The key is to choose your fats wisely. Overall, you should reduce saturated fats to less than 7 percent of total calories, avoid trans fats as much as possible, and incorporate heart-healthy polyunsaturated fats, including omega-3 fatty acids, and monounsaturated fats into your diet in moderation.

What about Cholesterol?

If you're like most people, cholesterol reduction is the first thing you think of in a heart-healthy diet. But, as you see from the discussion on fats, it's really more complex than looking at the amount of cholesterol in a particular food. Remember, cholesterol can be made by our bodies, as well as consumed through animal-based foods. Plants do not contain cholesterol. So, if you're eating a diet high in meat, poultry, and dairy products, such as butter and cheese, your diet is probably high in cholesterol. However, since your body makes cholesterol from both saturated and trans fats, it's best to look at the overall picture instead of focusing on dietary cholesterol. If you cut down on saturated and trans fats and replace them with polyunsaturated and monounsaturated fats, it's likely that you'll also be reducing your cholesterol intake.

Many of my patients ask me about consuming eggs when they are watching their cholesterol. Studies show that eating one egg per day does not lead to elevated cholesterol levels in healthy individuals, which means most people can eat eggs in moderation as part of a balanced diet. Again, it's the type and amount of fats you eat that contribute to unhealthy levels of cholesterol. Since the two go hand-in-hand, you'll find that most low-fat diets also limit cholesterol.

The bottom line on cholesterol: Guidelines recommend we limit our intake of cholesterol to less than 300 mg per day. The amount of cholesterol in packaged foods can be found on nutritional labels, while the amount of cholesterol in meat is listed on many web sites and online food diaries, and may also be provided by your physician.

Diet Staples—Protein and Carbs

Protein For most of us, the major components of our diets are protein and carbohydrates. Protein can come from either plants or animals and is a necessary part of every cell, tissue, and organ in our body. While we need some protein, most people consume much more than our bodies require. Recommended daily guidelines suggest that a woman age 19 to 70+ should have 46 grams of protein each day (growing children and athletes require slightly more). To put that into perspective, a three-ounce piece of meat contains 21 grams of protein.

The typical American diet is very high in animal-based proteins, particularly red meat. Eating red meat in moderaton is not a big "no-no." However, red meat can have a fair share of saturated fat and, depending on how it's prepared, also salt. When it comes to a heart-healthy diet, choosing lean meats (and eating them in moderation) is best. In addition, selecting alternative sources of protein can further reduce your risk for heart disease and stroke. As we discussed earlier, fish is a great protein choice—it's low in saturated fat and high in omega-3 fatty acids. Other good protein sources include:

- legumes (beans and peas)
- eggs (substitute egg whites if you're watching cholesterol intake)
- nuts and seeds
- low-fat dairy products, such as milk and yogurt

While there seems to be a high-protein diet craze lately, I would caution women not to follow such a restrictive eating plan. As I said, most people already consume more protein than necessary, and depending on the protein choices, such a diet could exceed guidelines for fat and cholesterol. Also, these diets can shortchange you on important whole grains, which, as we'll see in the next section, provide heart-healthy fiber and other valuable nutrients. A balanced diet is your best bet.

The bottom line on protein: Adult women should aim for 46 grams of protein per day. Choose lean protein sources, which are low in saturated fat.

Carbohydrates For years, cardiologists focused on reducing fats in the diet. It's only recently that we realized the important role carbohydrates play in our heart health. But, as with fats, not all carbohydrates are created equal. Basically, there are two types of carbohydrates: simple and complex. Simple carbohydrates include sugars that are found naturally in some foods, as well as sugar added during processing (e.g., cakes, cookies, candy, soda, and cereals with added sugar). Products made with refined or enriched (white) flour are also examples of simple carbs. These foods are converted quickly and easily into glucose (sugar) in the body and, therefore, cause spikes in blood sugar—not to mention that they are usually high in calories and have very little nutritional value.

Complex carbs, on the other hand, require more time and energy for the body to break down into fuel, which keeps blood sugar at a more consistent level and provides long-lasting energy for our bodies. Foods such as whole grains, fruits, and vegetables are examples of complex carbohydrates. Most people who have diabetes know all about "counting carbs"—they are looking for how the carbohydrate will break down and affect blood sugar. But, this is also important for the rest of us. Consuming complex carbohydrates can help you regulate blood sugar and, therefore, reduce your risk of developing diabetes and high blood pressure.

By eating whole grain foods and other complex carbs, you are also increasing your intake of fiber, and fiber is good for the body. Not only does fiber help regulate blood sugar, it aids in digestion, keeps our colons healthy, makes us feel fuller, and helps lower cholesterol. You've probably seen advertisements touting the cholesterol-lowering benefits of oat bran and oatmeal. Well, it's true—eating 10 to 25 grams of fiber each day can lower cholesterol by 10 percent.

Most of us do not get enough fiber in our diets. Many dietary guidelines suggest 25 or more grams of fiber per day, while the recent European Prevention Guidelines (presented in August 2012) along with the American Institute in Medicine recommend 30 to 45 grams of fiber per day for adults. Try recording the amount of fiber you eat in an average day. I suspect your total will be far less than these recommendations! The amount of fiber in a packaged food can be found in the nutritional information. You can easily obtain information on fiber for other foods, such as fruits and vegetables, online.

The research on carbohydrates is actually far more complicated. However, when I'm grocery shopping after a long day at work, I want simple rules to live by! When choosing carbs, keep these tips in mind:

- Load up on fruits and vegetables
- Buy whole grain breads, cereal, and pasta (make sure the food is labeled "whole" in the ingredients list). As you're reading the label, look for products with 5 or more grams of fiber per serving.
- Include other whole grain, high-fiber foods in your diet, such as brown rice, couscous, quinoa, lentils, beans, nuts and seeds, oat bran, and oatmeal.
- Avoid refined flour products and foods with added sugar, such as white bread, white rice, cakes, cookies, sugar-added cereals, and soda. Keep in mind that ingredients such as corn syrup, high-fructose corn syrup, dextrose, fructose, and corn sweetener, among others, are really sugar.

The bottom line on carbs and fiber: Choose complex carbs over simple carbs. Increase your dietary fiber to at least 25 grams per day by including whole grain foods at each meal. The term "whole grain" refers to grains that are minimally processed and have all the parts of the grain seed or kernel, including the bran, the germ, and the endosperm.

Fruits and Vegetables—Nature's Secret Weapon

Your mother was right: you should eat your vegetables and your fruit! Research shows that people who eat several servings of fruits and vegetables each day are at a lower risk for heart disease and stroke. Additionally, a diet high in fruits and vegetables has been linked to the prevention of certain types of cancer and can help you maintain a healthy weight. Because they are so beneficial, most guidelines recommend five or more daily servings of fruits and vegetables.

Not only do fruits and vegetables provide another valuable source of fiber, which lowers cholesterol, they are unmatched for supplying our bodies with a wide range of essential nutrients, including heart-healthy antioxidants. From beta-carotene, which protects our vision, to potassium, which helps keep blood pressure under control, fruits and vegetables are nature's vitamin powerhouse. Currently, there is no evidence that ingesting these vitamins in supplement form can reduce cardiovascular problems, but we know they are highly beneficial when eaten naturally. Therefore, the best way to get your vitamins is through the foods you eat (it's also much tastier).

To ensure you are getting a good variety of vitamins and antioxidants, make your meals colorful. Try eating fruits and veg-etables in a range of hues—red berries and grapes, green broccoli and spinach, purple eggplant, orange carrots and citrus fruits, and yellow pears and squash, to name just a few. While the typical dinner plate in the United States is rather bland in color (think meat and potatoes), a heart-healthy plate is like a rainbow.

The bottom line on fruits and vegetables: Aim for at least five servings of fruits and vegetables each day by including them in every meal and snacking on them in between. Adding fruit to your cereal, substituting vegetables for meat, tossing veggies with pasta, grabbing fruit for a snack, and enjoying a smoothie made with fruits and/or vegetables are just a few ways to increase your consumption.

The Sodium Factor

As mentioned in the chapter on blood pressure, I often find myself discussing sodium intake with my patients. Sodium (salt) is a major contributor to hypertension, and most of us consume too much of it. In fact, if you compare similar foods produced in different countries, you'll find that Americans have some of the saltiest fare in the world! Because sodium is added to so many of our foods, and we've become accustomed to eating a diet high in sodium, we don't recognize them as tasting salty. That's why many patients who go on a low-sodium diet have so much trouble adjusting in the beginning. They complain that food tastes bland. However, over time, as their taste buds adjust and they learn to enhance dishes with herbs and spices instead of salt, many find that food has much more flavor.

While a typical American diet has a sodium content of about 10 grams per day, current guidelines recommend adults over 51 years old consume only 1.5 grams or less per day. That's a significant difference. There is no doubt that a high-sodium diet puts you at increased risk for developing hypertension and stroke. The good news is that even a modest decrease in salt can reduce your blood pressure. To learn more about how to reduce sodium in your diet, as well as the results of a major study on sodium called DASH, please refer to chapter 6.

If I had to pick two things to focus on that relate to a heart-healthy diet, it would be increasing fiber and reducing sodium. Fiber can help reduce cholesterol, while sodium reduction lowers blood pressure—both major contributors to cardiovascular health.

Something to Drink with Your Meal?

We can't discuss diet without including beverages. Over the past several decades, the quantity of soft drinks (or soda) being consumed in America has skyrocketed. This is a source of empty calories and sugar that is contributing to epidemics of obesity and diabetes. Although soft drinks are not solely responsible, the increase in serving size that many of us drink is a major factor. Consider this: drinking two regular servings (about 12 ounces each) of a sweetened beverage per day can increase your risk of heart disease by approximately 35 percent. A 20-ounce bottle of cola has over 60 grams of sugar and more than 250 calories!

While diet beverages are low in calories, they are still not a good choice. Diet beverages have not been associated with an increased risk for heart disease, but they have been linked to metabolic syndrome or prediabetes. Juice may be a slightly better option, but calories and sugar can still be a factor. I counsel my patients, particularly those who are trying to lose weight, that eating a piece of fruit, which provides fiber, is more beneficial and filling than drinking juice.

Though it may not seem exciting, water is the best option for hydration. Not only is it free of calories and sugar, it's essential for your body. In many parts of the world, safe drinking water is a luxury. However, here in the United States, we have no excuse.

If you want to spice things up, you can try flavored water or add fresh fruit, such as lemon, lime, or orange to your glass.

Alcohol

When discussing heart disease, many women ask me about alcohol and its effects. There is some evidence to suggest that moderate alcohol consumption is associated with a decreased risk for heart disease and stroke. Red wine, in particular, contains polyphenols (such as reservatrol) found in the skin of the grapes, which have been linked to heart health. Other types of alcohol have also been associated with a lower risk of heart disease, although the precise scientific reasons are still unclear. It may be that alcohol helps to increase HDL cholesterol slightly. Regardless of the reason, the key word is *moderate*. For women, this means one drink equal to 5 ounces of wine, 12 ounces of beer, or 1.5 ounces of liquor per day.

Of course, excessive drinking of alcohol is never a good idea. Too much alcohol can lead to high blood pressure, liver damage, atrial fibrillation of the heart, and even a weakening of the heart muscle called cardiomyopathy. In addition, studies suggest that women who drink alcohol are at an increased risk for breast cancer. You should also ask your physician if drinking alcohol is safe for you. Many medications do not interact well with alcohol, which means you may need to abstain from it altogether.

Vitamins and Other Supplements

To fill in the gaps of a balanced diet, many people reach for a pill. Millions of people also take vitamins and other supplements in an effort to reduce their risk of heart disease and stroke. Because supplements are considered food, they are not regulated as medications. Over time, large-scale studies have not demonstrated a benefit for the majority of vitamins and supplements being consumed. Taking vitamins A and E, for instance, has not been associated with a reduction in heart attacks and strokes. Other vitamins, such as B vitamins and vitamin C, which have been thought to reduce heart disease and stroke due to their status as antioxidants, have not been proven beneficial in supplement form. Therefore, current guidelines do not recommend these vitamins for use in cardiovascular disease prevention.

Currently, vitamin D is being studied in a large randomized control trial. It will be interesting to see whether this vitamin reduces the risk for heart disease, since smaller studies have suggested this may be the case. Since large numbers of people do have vitamin D deficiencies, an association with heart disease would have significant public health implications.

When it comes to vitamins and other supplements, it's really "buyer beware." There are hundreds of supplements available at your local store, as well as over the Internet, but the majority of these products have not been well studied. Package labels may not be accurate, and information on potential side effects is often limited or nonexistent. This doesn't mean the benefits of vitamins and other natural remedies do not exist; it simply means we have a long way to go in knowing exactly what those benefits are and how to make the most of them. Before you spend your hard-earned money on a supplement, do a little research of your own. The National Institutes of Health has a special section called the National Center for Complementary and Alternative Medicine (NCCAM) that examines alternative therapies. The NCCAM also has an excellent web site with information on vitamins and supplements. Likewise, you can ask your health-care provider about what may be right for you. (See the Resources section for more information.)

The Big Picture

Now that we've looked at specific dietary components, let's talk about the bigger picture. In the United States and most industrialized countries, too many of us are overweight or obese—an estimated two-thirds of U.S. adults fall into this category. This increase in weight, which has occurred over the past several decades and is related to changes in the way we live, is having a major impact on our health. As we discussed in the last chapter, modern conveniences have made daily exercise nearly nonexistent. You can also blame the prevalence of fast, cheap food that is calorie dense and high in fat. Finally, portion sizes have expanded just like our waistlines.

As a population, we need to make some changes. Recently, I have been encouraged to see the beginnings of such change. Health policies that urge food manufacturers and restaurants to make healthy modifications, as well as provide information on calories, sodium, and fat content, are steps in the right direction. School wellness programs that focus on improving nutrition and nutritional education for our children are also fantastic. However, until we, as individuals, alter our dietary patterns, we will not see real improvements in our health.

Women are in a unique position to lead a revolution in healthy eating! As women, we are still primarily responsible for purchasing groceries and preparing meals, which means we can impact not only our own health, but the health of those around us. By simply choosing whole grains, filling up your cart with more fruits and vegetables, buying leaner proteins, and stocking up on healthy choices for last-minute meals (frozen veggies and brown rice, for example), you can make a significant difference.

I am also a big believer in slowing down when it comes to

mealtime. Preparing and sharing meals together can empower everyone to make healthy choices. Families who eat meals together not only reinforce healthy behaviors, but also benefit from the time spent together. In today's hectic world, this can be difficult to do. Try setting aside just one or two days a week to prepare and eat a meal together. Making meals in advance can also reduce stress (and temptation) on busy nights. (See "Simple Strategies for Heart-Healthy Eating" for more tips.)

A Note about Weight Loss

Many women are interested in losing weight, particularly as they get older. As we age, we tend to lose lean muscle and gain fat. Keeping a healthy weight—with a body mass index of less than 25 kg/m^2—is important for heart health, as well as preventing diabetes and hypertension. Entire books are written about weight loss, so I would rather focus on the key aspects of a healthy diet. The components we've already discussed—a diet high in fiber, fruits, and vegetables and low in saturated fats and refined sugar—will assist with weight loss, if needed. Reducing portion sizes and increasing physical activity can also help you maintain a healthy weight. In other words, what's good for heart health is also good for weight management.

I would like to mention a few other tips that may help with weight management. First, weighing yourself periodically can keep you on track. It's amazing how those extra pounds can sneak up on you! If you see that you are gaining a couple of pounds, you can cut back on the extras. On the flip side, weighing yourself every day can be discouraging. Instead of worrying about your day-to-day weight (which tends to fluctuate naturally), try weighing yourself once a week or simply focusing on how your clothes fit. When things start to feel snug, it's time to make some changes.

Online food diaries are also beneficial. Being more aware of the calorie and nutritional content of the foods you eat can help you make healthier choices. Some of these diaries offer free phone apps, allowing you to take them wherever you go.

Finally, eating breakfast may be a key factor in weight management. Investigators found that men and women who had lost over 30 pounds and kept it off a year or more were more likely to eat breakfast every day. The participants were also more apt to check their weight regularly and modify their behaviors if they noticed an increase.

As I'm sure you know, there is no magic solution for weight loss. Many women feel as though they are constantly struggling with weight issues. However, the healthy choices you make for your heart can also help you win the weight loss battle.

Simple Strategies for Heart-Healthy Eating

Mealtime should be a low-key, relaxed time of the day—not one in which we feel guilt with every bite. Food shopping should also be stress free. We have enough to worry about in our daily lives. Fortunately, eating a heart-healthy diet doesn't have to be complicated. With a few simple strategies, you can make mealtimes easier and healthier.

Get Family and Friends Involved

- Making both shopping and meal preparation a family affair is a great way to keep yourself on track, as well as model healthy behaviors. If you have children, get them involved by planning meals together. At our house, my sons help me create a meal plan for the week ahead. We use this meal plan as a grocery list, which cuts down on time in the store. Having a plan also reduces stress after a busy day at work, since we're not at a loss for dinner ideas (and less tempted to order a pizza!).

- Another way to get the kids involved is by having them assist in the kitchen. When my sons were younger, I kept a step stool near the sink so they could help wash fruits and vegetables and mix ingredients. Children who participate in meal preparation are more likely to eat what they've helped create, as well as learn about healthy food choices.

- If you're on your own, try hosting a once-a-month potluck dinner to try new heart-healthy recipes. Not only is it a great way to sample something new, it's a good excuse to spend time with friends!

Be Prepared

- Having a meal plan is one way to cut down on stress and temptation during the week. Another way is to prepare meals in advance. Spend a Sunday afternoon with family or friends cooking a few healthy meals for the week ahead. Making a large batch of soup that can be shared, or roasting a whole chicken that can be used in several recipes, will save both time and money—and it's a nice way to spend time together.

- When you bring fruit and veggies home, spend some time washing and cutting them up into easy-to-grab portions. You're more likely to snack on carrot sticks if they're already prepared. I like to cut up oranges and leave them on the counter just before or after dinner. It makes the choice of having fruit for a snack or dessert a little easier for everyone.

- To beat the morning rush, have the kids pack their lunches the night before. Bringing lunch to school is not only healthier, it will save you money. It's also a great teaching opportunity. Have kids build a healthy lunch by including one lean protein (meat or low-fat dairy), 1–2 whole grains, and 1–2 fruits and/or vegetables. You can lead by example by packing your own healthy lunch!

Control Portions

- Studies have shown that using smaller plates can reduce the number of calories consumed. At home, try using smaller plates for your meals. Then, think of your plate as a pie chart. One quarter should be a lean protein (about the size of your fist or a deck of cards). Another quarter should be a whole-grain selection, and the other half of your plate should be filled with vegetables or fruit. Salad plates are another story—bigger is better. Just be sure to measure out the salad dressing.
- When eating out, try asking for a "to go" container at the beginning of your meal. Before you begin eating, divide your meal in half and put it in the container. With only half a portion on your plate, you won't be tempted to eat the entire meal (which is typically too large at restaurants). Or, you can split a meal with a friend or family member. Having a salad along with half of the main entrée will likely fill you up.
- Don't be afraid to ask for salad dressing on the side, or to substitute a salad or a vegetable for fries. Also, many restaurants will swap brown rice (a healthy whole grain) for white rice or less healthy starches such as pasta or potatoes, if you request it.

To download a free shopping companion guide and list of some great healthy products to try, visit www.sprypubdiet.com. Good eating!

Take a Step

Changing your eating habits can seem overwhelming, but like any change, it gets easier over time. Reading labels, planning healthy meals, and learning new recipes take more effort in the beginning, but as you become more familiar with good food choices, these changes will become routine. And, once you start feeling the benefits of a healthy diet, you'll be encouraged to continue. The results are gratifying: with a healthy diet you can reduce cholesterol levels in as little as four weeks.

I advise my patients to take small, steady steps toward healthy eating. Try incorporating just one of the dietary guidelines we've covered, such as increasing fiber or lowering sodium, each month. Then, add another. Each day you can choose to do something positive, whether it's reducing portion sizes or forgoing that soda. Just remember that adopting a healthy diet is not a short-term fix—it's a commitment to eating better for life!

CHAPTER TWELVE

Get Moving

The only thing that makes my heart beat faster than running a marathon is a great shoe sale.

ANONYMOUS

I suspect you already know that exercise is good for you. Most Americans do. Yet, according to surveys only 40 percent of adults in the United States meet the minimum physical activity requirements for heart health—at least two and a half hours of moderate physical activity a week or 30 minutes each day. That's worrisome because physical inactivity is a major risk factor for cardiovascular problems. In fact, being sedentary can double the threat for developing heart disease, while adults who exercise regularly have about a 40 percent lower risk for heart disease or stroke compared to those who do not.

It's not just your heart that will benefit from regular exercise. You can reduce your chances of developing many chronic health issues, including nearly all the major risk factors for heart disease, by stepping up your activity level. Regular exercise can help:

- **Control your weight**—Lack of regular physical activity increases the likelihood of becoming overweight or obese, which can lead to diabetes, hypertension, and high cholesterol, among other potential health problems.

- **Lower your blood pressure**—Regular exercise can lower blood pressure by about 5 to 15 mmHg, which can mean the difference between having to take a medication to lower blood pressure or not.
- **Regulate blood sugar**—Exercise improves your body's ability to regulate blood sugar, lessening your resistance to insulin. Increasing muscle mass and decreasing fat help your body to use insulin more effectively. For folks with a family history of diabetes or those who meet the criteria for metabolic syndrome, exercise is critical for preventing diabetes. As you may recall from chapter 8, a large-scale study comparing lifestyle factors (including exercise) with the use of medication to control blood sugar found that lifestyle changes were more successful than prescription drugs in the prevention of diabetes.
- **Improve cholesterol levels**—We also know that lack of regular physical activity affects your cholesterol in a negative way. Conversely, regular exercise can keep harmful triglycerides and LDL cholesterol levels low, while boosting levels of heart-healthy HDL cholesterol.
- **Reduce inflammation**—Studies show that regular physical activity reduces inflammation in the body, which, in turn, decreases your risk for heart disease. Adults who exercise display lower levels of C-reactive protein, a marker of inflammation.
- **Lessen symptoms of depression/anxiety and reduce chronic stress**—By stimulating chemicals in the brain that leave you feeling happier and more relaxed, exercise can boost your mood. There is ample evidence that regular exercise reduces

anxiety and stress and can lessen the symptoms of depression—improving your quality of life, as well as protecting your heart.

- **Support other healthy changes**—Studies show that exercise can help smokers kick the habit by reducing nicotine cravings and providing an outlet for nervous energy. By the same token, exercise can also reduce food cravings for those who are making dietary changes.

How Exercise Affects the Heart

The heart is a muscle, and like all muscles, it needs regular exercise to keep it fit. When you are inactive, the heart muscle gets weaker, and a weak heart pumps less blood with each beat than a strong heart. Because a lower volume of blood is being pumped into the circulatory system, the heart has to beat more often to ensure proper circulation to all areas of the body. A consistently rapid heartbeat not only puts more strain on the heart, it may result in higher blood pressure over time, which can cause hardening of the arteries. In contrast, a fit heart will have a slower resting heart rate and produce more robust circulation, keeping artery walls in good condi-

Recommendations from the American Heart Association/American College of Cardiology (and the American College of Sports Medicine) specify 30 minutes of moderate activity most days of the week (give or more) or 20 minutes of vigorous activity three or more days per week. In general, that's about 150 minutes of moderate activity or 75 minutes of vigorous activity per week. If you need to lose weight, often this amount of exercise is not enough. In addition to aerobic exercise, current guidelines also recommend adding activities that help with flexibility, balance, and strength. This is particularly important for women, who are at risk for developing osteoporosis and need flexibility, balance, and strength for fall prevention.

tion. Exercise also delivers oxygen and nutrients to your tissues, which helps the cardiovascular system work more efficiently.

In addition to keeping your heart strong and reducing blood pressure, regular exercise affects many other cardiac risk factors, as we've learned. By helping your body regulate blood sugar levels, it decreases your chances of developing insulin resistance and diabetes. Exercise also contributes to a healthy cholesterol profile by lowering LDL and triglyceride levels, and increasing HDL or good cholesterol. It helps you burn more calories, which leads to better weight management and less inflammation in the body. All of this reduces your risk of heart disease.

Fitness is so important to your heart that it may be a better predictor of serious cardiovascular events than EKG (electrocardiogram) results. A study of almost 3,000 women who underwent a cardiac stress test found that EKG changes (which were mild) were not predictive of death due to cardiovascular disease, while exercise capacity was a reliable indicator. When I order a stress test for a patient, one of the key factors I look at is her ability to exercise. If she has poor exercise tolerance, which is an indicator of poor fitness, I know her risk for heart disease is

The Nurses' Health Study, which followed a large group of women for several decades, looked at the benefits of physical activity, including brisk walking. The study found that walking lowers your risk for heart disease. And the benefits were similar no matter what weight the subject was, which means that being overweight does not negate the gains of improving your fitness level. Even those women who started exercising later in life (midlife or older) saw health improvements. These researchers also observed that while light exercise was heart healthy, the longer the exercise was performed, the greater the benefit. For example, walking two or more hours per week lowered the risk for heart disease by more than 50 percent.

increased, even if all the other components of the test are normal.

Aging or Inactivity?

It's interesting to note that many of the problems we've come to associate with normal aging, such as loss of strength, balance, and flexibility, are not necessarily a natural consequence of getting older. Research indicates that many of these issues are a result of years of inactivity, which means we can often improve our quality of life as we age by getting more exercise. Even cognitive function can be improved with regular exercise, lessening our chances of developing memory loss or dementia in later years.

The time to start is now! As we've discussed, our modern culture has reduced the need for physical activity and led to a sedentary lifestyle for most of us. Today in the United States, our adolescents and young adults are more likely to be overweight than ever before, increasing their risk for diabetes and high cholesterol. Because of this, population trends suggest that younger men and women have greater risks for heart disease. Conversely, studies show that women (and men) age 30 or younger who are physically fit are much less likely to have prediabetes, diabetes, hypertension, and unhealthy cholesterol profiles compared to younger adults who are inactive.

Alas, exercise is not the fountain of youth; it won't prevent every ailment that comes with getting older. However, research shows it can stave off many health problems, including heart disease, and therefore improve the aging process. According to the American Heart Association, for every hour of regular exercise you perform, you'll gain about two hours of additional life expectancy. And, by warding off health problems, exercise can not only add years to your life, it can add life to your years!

Exercise for Older Women

Starting to exercise at an early age is important, but it's never too late to improve your health. No matter what your age or physical abilities, regular exercise is beneficial—even if you have a history of heart disease and/or stroke. Research confirms that people who are physically active after a first heart attack or stroke have a significantly lower risk of a second cardiac event when compared to people who remained inactive.

Of course, it's important to talk with your physician before starting any exercise program. If you've had a heart attack or stroke, there may be limitations to what you can do, particularly in the short term. Participation in a cardiac rehabilitation program can help you develop an exercise routine that is right for you, while being carefully monitored. These programs set individual goals in terms of activities, duration, heart rate, and blood pressure, based on your health condition. Many studies have found that participation in a cardiac rehab program lowers the risk for future heart attack and can be especially beneficial for older women. (See chapter 2 for more on cardiac rehab.)

It's no secret that as women age, we tend to gain weight and lose muscle mass. Regular physical activity is imperative to prevent both, while keeping our hearts strong. You don't have to be young and healthy, or a super athlete, to reap the benefits of exercise. Walking is something most people can do regardless of age. Even if you are physically limited, there is some type of activity that can be incorporated into your daily routine. Remember that something is always better than nothing! If you are feeling overwhelmed or confused about what type of exercise you can do, try consulting your health-care provider or a physical therapist. In other words, there's no excuse not to get moving.

Visit the American Heart Association web site to learn about exercise tips for older adults.

How Much Activity Is Enough?

The American Heart Association recommends at least two and a half hours of moderate physical activity per week, which translates into approximately 30 minutes per day, five days a week. Of course, more is better! In general, moderate-intensity exercise is defined as any activity that causes your heart rate and breathing pattern to noticeably increase. You should still be able to carry on a conversation, but not be able to sing.

More specifically, the Centers for Disease Control defines moderate intensity as exercising at 50 to 70 percent of your maximum heart rate, which is roughly calculated as 220 minus your age. This number represents the upper limit of what your cardiovascular system can handle during physical activity. However, this calculation is an estimate that provides an average value. Many people have a higher or lower maximum heart rate, depending on their fitness level and overall health. For this reason, your heart rate, which is expressed in beats per minute (bpm) is typically expressed as a range, rather than a specific number. In general, a healthy 49-year-old woman has a maximum recommended heart rate of 220 − 49 = 171 bpm—70 percent of her maximum heart rate would be approximately 120 bpm, which is her target for a moderate-intensity workout. You can find heart rate calculators on many web sites, including www.mayoclinic.com and www.active.com.

The good news is you don't need expensive equipment or a gym membership to fulfill these requirements. Walking briskly for 30 minutes (approximately two miles at a pace of 4.0 mph) or bicycling for five miles in 30 minutes is considered moderate activity. There are many other activities to choose from, including 30 minutes of water aerobics, swimming laps for 20 minutes, playing volleyball for 45 minutes, and even participating in wheelchair basketball for 20 minutes. The key is to find an activity, or preferably several activities, that you enjoy and can participate in regularly.

You can also break up your exercise routine into smaller time slots. Accumulating three ten-minute stretches of exercise throughout the day still meets the minimum requirements for heart health. So, for instance, you can take a brisk ten-minute morning walk and then go on a 20-minute bike ride later in the evening. It all adds up!

If you have been sedentary and are just starting an exercise routine, don't be discouraged if you are unable to meet the recommendations right away. Just do what you can and build slowly. For example, try walking for ten minutes at a slower pace every day. After a week, add five minutes more to your walk and pick up the pace a bit. Before you know it, you'll be at the recommended level. The important thing is to keep moving.

Developing the Exercise Habit

Several years ago, I conducted a survey of doctors in training, along with those of us who had completed training, regarding exercise habits. Not surprisingly, I found that even many physicians don't get enough exercise! Like you, we lead very busy lives, which can make finding time for exercise a challenge. But that doesn't mean we should give up. Because physical activity is so important for our health and well-being, we need to make it a priority—even if we have to get creative about how we incorporate it into our daily lives.

Often, the first thing we need to do is change our attitude toward exercise. If we think about exercising for a specific period, such as 30 or 60 minutes, we might decide we don't have time and do nothing at all. But, as we've seen, even smaller bouts of exercise can make a difference. When you watch young children at play, you find they are often stopping and starting activities; they're not worrying about the duration of an activity, but simply having fun. As adults, too often we are focused on a specific outcome and missing that sense of fun. So, why not think of exercise as playing instead of a chore? Try a new activity. Challenge yourself. Find a sport or class you take pleasure in. Being active should be enjoyable. And, don't let worrying about whether you're in good enough shape or if you'll excel at something stop you from trying. Everyone needs to start somewhere.

You're more likely to develop a habit of exercising if you think of it as fun rather than a chore. Have you always wanted to try ballroom dancing? Does the local community center offer water aerobics? Do you have a friend who might like to take a yoga class with you? Trying new activities and being creative can help keep you motivated and connect with family and friends. For instance, a neighborhood walking club combines social interaction with fitness. Getting the kids off the couch for a nature hike or a game of football not only counts as exercise, it's an opportunity to spend time together. Make exercise something you look forward to.

It's also helpful to set a goal when you start to increase your physical activity. It should be a realistic, achievable goal, but one that keeps you on track. Something as simple as walking 20 minutes every day is a good place to start. Unless you define what you're trying to accomplish, it can be difficult to gauge your progress.

Social support is another great way to ensure your success. You may not be the type of person who likes to exercise in a group, but having a friend, spouse, or child as an exercise partner can provide motivation and make it harder to skip. I like going to the gym with my sons. We don't work out together, but they help keep me on track. If I had to go alone at the end of a long day, I might easily think of several reasons not to do it!

I also use a calendar as a reminder, which helps push me out of inertia. Every day that I exercise, I put a big "X" over that date. Since the calendar is by the door, I see it every time I enter the house. It can really start to bother me if I see a bunch of days with no Xs. Finding a visible reminder that works for you can be a good motivator. There are many online exercise diaries that can track your exercise habits and even send you text or email reminders. Many of these apps now use social media components to provide a supportive community.

It's also a good idea to take a look at your past exercise habits. What motivated you to exercise, and what created barriers or made you stop? If you've never been very active, you can start by writing down a list of activities you would consider trying, and then commit to one. If you find that your schedule gets in the way, block out time slots (in ink!) in your calendar and treat these as you would any other important appointment. Most people find packing a gym bag and going right from work better than going home first, where it's easy to get sidetracked. The key is finding what works for you and sticking with it.

Finally, don't discount the amount of exercise you get just from your daily activities. While this type of exercise does not count toward the recommendations for heart health, it does provide benefits. Wearing a pedometer or some other tracking device can reveal how many steps you take in the course of a day, and may help you stay motivated. Aim for approximately 10,000 steps per day, which is the equivalent of about five miles. You might be surprised by how much (or perhaps, how little) you move during the day. If the number is lower than you'd like, you can sneak more exercise into your daily routine by trying these tips:

- Take your athletic shoes to work and include a ten-minute walk in your lunch break.
- Instead of sending an email, get up and go talk to a coworker face-to-face.
- When running errands, park as far from the entrance as possible.
- Stand up and pace around when talking on the phone instead of sitting.
- Get up from your desk once every hour and walk somewhere. (Set a timer if you need to.)
- Ride your bike or walk to complete an errand instead of driving.
- Play outdoor games with your children instead of watching television.
- If you're watching television, get up during the commercials and stretch or do a few crunches.
- Rake leaves instead of using a leaf blower.
- Make housework a workout.
- Use the stairs instead of the elevator whenever possible.

The benefits of regular exercise are hard to ignore. In addition to improving heart health, you may find that increasing your activity level gives you more energy, helps you sleep better, and even boosts your self-confidence. Believe me, I know it can be difficult to add one more thing to an already busy schedule, but when you consider what an important role exercise plays in our health, doesn't it deserve priority in our lives? You can't wait until your schedule is better, because there is never an ideal time. If you're just starting a family, it's hard to squeeze in regular exercise around caring for young children. If you're busy with a career, long hours can put a crimp in your exercise routine. As you get older, health issues may get in the way of being active. But keep in mind, there are many people out there with child-care responsibilities, demanding jobs, or physical limitations who are finding time to exercise. And, you can do it, too! Get started today by:

- **Consulting with your health-care provider**—This is a good place to start if you haven't been exercising. Make sure you're healthy enough for the activity you have chosen. He or she can also help you design an exercise plan that is right for your individual goals/needs.

- **Setting a goal**—It's easy to say you'll exercise every day, but you're more likely to do it if you have a specific goal. Write it down and put it in a visible location. Better yet, schedule it on your calendar.

- **Getting prepared**—Buy yourself a good pair of athletic shoes and keep them in a convenient location. If you're planning on walking outside, make sure you're outfitted for changing weather conditions. If you're using a treadmill, find music, television shows, or books that you enjoy while ticking off the miles.

- **Being creative**—Sign up for an exercise class. Yoga and Pilates are great for increasing balance, strength, and flexibility, while high-energy dance or aerobics classes offer good cardio workouts. Team sports for adults can be a fun way to meet people and stay in shape. You might try organizing a neighborhood walking club or simply enlisting a friend to join you for a daily walk. Find what appeals to you.

- **Just doing it**—Like the famous tagline says … just do it. Find 10 to 20 minutes today to take a walk, ride a bike, or play soccer with the kids. The more you get moving, the easier it becomes.

CHAPTER THIRTEEN

The Stress Factor

The purpose of stress isn't to hurt you, but to let you know it's time to go back to the heart and start loving.

SARA PADDISON, *The Hidden Power of the Heart*

We've all heard the amazing stories about mothers who seem to develop superhuman strength as they rush in to save a child from a life-threatening situation. Afterward, they marvel at their ability to lift a heavy object or move with surprising speed without even thinking about it. When faced with danger, we all have the capacity to become superheroes, thanks to a natural physiological response often referred to as the "fight or flight" response—it's also known as stress. Though we tend to associate stress with tension, anxiety, and other negative emotions, it can actually save your life in an emergency. The problem with stress occurs when it becomes chronic and unmanaged. In that case, stress can be very harmful to our bodies, especially our hearts.

The Stress Response

Let's say you're driving on the highway and a car suddenly veers in front of you, almost causing a collision. As you react to this dangerous scenario, your body responds in several ways. First, two powerful neurotransmitters (chemicals that carry messages to and from your nerves) called epinephrine (adrenaline) and norepinephrine are released by your adrenal gland. Meanwhile, your pituitary gland, located at the base of the brain, secretes hormones, including cortisol. These neurochemicals and hormones prepare you for action by prompting your heart to pump more oxygen-rich blood throughout your body, which increases your heart rate and your blood pressure. While relaxing arteries to allow more blood flow to the brain and large muscle groups (both vital in a threatening situation), this surge of chemicals restricts arteries in other areas of the body, such as your digestive system. In addition, extra blood sugar is released into the bloodstream to provide a boost of energy. Your breathing becomes more rapid, perspiration levels increase, and your senses are heightened—all of which is cleverly designed to help you respond effectively in an emergency.

Stress is unavoidable; but it's how we respond to the challenges and difficulties we confront every day that determines the effects of stress on our health. In large part, our ability to cope with stress is based on internal factors, such as proper nutrition, fitness level, emotional well-being, sufficient sleep, and overall health. If you are feeling overwhelmed by stress, taking better care of yourself is an important step in managing those feelings.

Once the threat of danger is gone and you begin to relax, the stress response subsides, returning your bodily functions to a normal state. But what if the stress response stays active? In today's world, the stress response is often triggered when there is no immediate physical danger, but rather during a constant barrage of mental or emotional pressures. Tight work deadlines, a hectic commute, too many family obligations, financial worries, health problems, caring for elderly parents, and feeling there is not enough time in a day to accomplish everything you need to do—these are the modern stressors that can take a toll on our health, if we let them.

We all experience stress, but for some people, stress levels stay consistently high, and therefore their bodies are continually bombarded by the effects of stress hormones. Over time, excessive levels of these chemicals can weaken the immune system and cause muscle tension and headaches, digestive problems, insomnia, and depression or anxiety, among other problems. Excessive levels of these hormones also increase your risk for cardiovascular disease.

How Stress Affects Your Heart

As we've seen, the hormones released during stressful situations can constrict blood vessels, rev up your heart rate, raise blood pressure, and increase blood sugar. If stress levels remain high over a prolonged period of time, these effects can cause damage to the vessels, which we know leads to the development of atherosclerosis and heart disease. Chronic stress also increases LDL (bad) cholesterol and triglyceride levels, while decreasing HDL (good) cholesterol, which, again, contributes to heart disease. Additionally, chronic stress produces inflammation in the body, which also elevates your risk for cardiac events, such as heart attacks.

Charles Mayo, MD, one of the founders of the Mayo Clinic said, "Worry and stress affect the circulation, the heart, the glands, the whole nervous system, and profoundly affects heart action."

Studies show that personality traits such as negativity and anger may also be linked to heart disease. It's easy to understand why—the spikes in blood sugar, elevated blood pressure, and other changes that occur when we experience negative emotions can be corrosive to our arteries. Similarly, depression is associated with an increased risk for heart attacks and cardiovascular death, as well. A large British study, which followed the cardiovascular health of over 19,000 men and women, found that those who suffered from depression were three times more likely to die from heart disease compared to participants who were not depressed, even after adjusting for other risk factors. This increased risk can be traced back to inflammation; individuals with depression are more likely to have elevated levels of inflammatory markers, such as C-reactive protein, which is a cardiac risk factor.

Since women have a higher rate of depression than men, this connection to heart health may be particularly important for us. Although it's not clear whether the treatment of depression reduces the incidence of heart disease, treatment does improve a patient's quality of life, and with the reduction of depressive symptoms, a person is more likely to participate in heart-healthy behaviors such as regular exercise and smoking cessation.

For women who have heart disease, reducing stress is even more important. When the heart is compromised, common stressors such as an argument or public speaking can put increased demands on the heart muscle, resulting in ischemia (a lack of blood flow to the heart) and chest pain or angina. After a heart attack, many patients feel increased levels of stress and often experience symptoms of depression and/or anxiety. Over the past several decades, health-care providers have begun to recognize the importance of managing these conditions in order to prevent future heart events. Although in many cases there is still a lack of resources and training to fully manage these conditions, I believe this is changing for the better. Today we see more facilities putting an emphasis on the psychosocial aspects of cardiac health, as well training health-care providers to properly treat these issues. If you have been diagnosed with heart disease or have had a heart attack, do not ignore the stress that often accompanies recovery. Seeking treatment for all aspects of your condition is important for heart health.

The Broken Heart Syndrome

While chronic stress has a cumulative effect—that is, the damage builds over time—acute stress can also affect the heart. A severe emotional event, such as the death of a loved one, a natural disaster, or even an extremely heated argument, can trigger a response that causes the heart to function abnormally, even to the point of mimicking a heart attack. When this happens, the left ventricular wall fails to move as well as it needs to, and the individual experiencing the stressful event may even have increases in troponin levels (troponins are a type of protein), which we see during a heart attack. Often during these episodes, the heart appears to balloon out at the bottom, which is called *takotsubo cardiomyopathy* or broken heart syndrome. (Takotsubo is the Japanese name for old-fashioned octopus traps, which is what the heart resembles in this situation.)

This stress-induced condition is more common in women than men and happens more often in post-menopausal women compared to premenopausal women. Symptoms of broken heart syndrome are similar to that of a heart attack, including chest pain and shortness of breath. Some women may even experience signs of heart failure. Because it so closely resembles a heart attack, the majority of women who experience this condition receive a coronary angiography to look for blockages in the artery, but typically none are found. Fortunately, this condition usually resolves over time—often a month or two. Patients may receive medications (the same ones used for heart attacks) to help relieve symptoms, and follow-up tests normally show dramatic improvement. Although data are limited, most experts believe the long-term prognosis is excellent. So, while you may not die from a broken heart, it can be very traumatic.

How Much Stress Is Too Much?

Our reaction to stress is highly individualized. While some women may thrive on a busy lifestyle, with a demanding job and a full calendar of activities, others are more content when life moves at a slightly slower pace. In addition, some people are more prone to the effects of stress than others. The symptoms of stress overload can manifest themselves in many ways, including:

Physical Symptoms
- sleep disturbances
- muscle tension and aches
- gastrointestinal problems, such as chronic indigestion and ulcers
- extreme fatigue
- headaches, including migraines

Emotional and Behavioral Symptoms
- anxiety and nervousness
- change in eating habits (i.e., loss of appetite or overeating)
- mood swings/irritability
- lack of enthusiasm/energy
- depression

In some cases, chronic stress can lead to unhealthy behaviors, such as alcohol and drug abuse or cigarette smoking, as a way to cope. Unfortunately, this type of behavior only makes matters worse. By altering your body chemicals, alcohol and drugs make small problems seem bigger than they really are, resulting in a greater and more prolonged stress response. And, because of the negative impacts these behaviors have on your overall health, you are less able to cope with stress, feeding the addiction and creating a vicious cycle.

The bottom line is that everyone has his or her own threshold for stress. If you are experiencing some of the symptoms listed above, you should talk to your health-care provider about ways to manage stress. A good physician will not dismiss your concerns regarding stress, but rather will be willing to listen and offer resources to help you cope.

Stress-Management Strategies

For most of us, stress is a daily component of life. The goal is not to eliminate all stress, which is virtually impossible, but to manage it effectively. Fortunately, the number of stress-reduction techniques and therapies available has grown over recent years. In addition to talking with your physician, there are some proven stress reduction techniques you can try on your own.

Identify Your Stress A good place to start is with some self-analysis. If you are feeling overly stressed, ask yourself these questions:
- When do I feel most stressed (i.e., a specific time of the day, during a specific activity)?
- Are there certain situations that make me feel more stressed?
- Am I overcommitted? Are there things I can say "no" to?
- Am I neglecting myself while taking caring of others?
- Do I have unrealistic expectations?
- Are there things I could ask others to help me with or provide support for?
- What triggers my anxiety?

A journal can be a useful tool when recording what makes you feel stressed out and, more importantly, what relieves your stress. Most often it's not just one situation or event, but rather the cumulative result of many pressures throughout your day that results in undue stress.

Now consider the flip side: ask yourself when your stress level is at its lowest—when you are feeling calm, relaxed, and in control of the situation. Is it a specific time of the day or during certain activities? What elements of this low-stress environment/activity can you use when stress levels are high? For example:

- Can you use music to relax at work or during your commute?
- Can you sit quietly and relax or meditate for five to ten minutes each day?
- Can you take a brisk ten-minute walk outside just prior to or after a stressful situation?

Be creative—try different things to help combat stress throughout the day. Be playful—have a good time as you experiment with stress-reduction techniques. Sing along or dance to your favorite music, spend a few minutes playing a word game, lose yourself in a good book, find a hobby that engrosses you, or make time to chat with a friend. Ask yourself: what gives me pleasure?—and then try to incorporate that activity into your life on a regular basis. This may not get rid of all your stress, but chances are your chronic stress level will decrease.

Of course, the most important question you need to ask is this: are the things you stress over more important than your health and well-being?

> While situations or events may seem stressful, it's how we perceive and react to these events that determine whether or not the stress response is activated. When you find yourself in a stressful situation, ask yourself if this will make a difference a year or five years from now. If it won't, then don't stress over it. If it will make a difference, then take action toward improving or changing the thing that is stressing you. In other words, by not letting stress control you, you are controlling your stress.

Probably not. Sometimes simply changing our attitudes or responses toward stressful situations can make all the difference.

Just Breathe Relaxation techniques such as deep breathing and meditation are powerful weapons against stress. Studies show that relaxation techniques can lower your heart rate, blood pressure, and blood glucose levels, as well as reduce pain and anxiety and improve healing. Though we continue to discover the benefits of these techniques, the research is not new. In the 1970s, Dr. Herbert Benson of Harvard University uncovered an antidote to the stress response, which he called the "relaxation response." The relaxation response is "a physical state of deep rest that changes the physical and emotional responses to stress, and the opposite of the fight or flight response." Participants in Dr. Benson's studies used transcendental meditation to decrease their heart rates and blood pressure, slow their rate of breathing, reduce muscle tension, and direct blood flow to their extremities. This strong connection between mind and body is used today to combat the negative effects of stress and aid in healing.

You needn't be an expert in relaxation techniques or a Zen master to benefit. Simply engaging in deep breathing exercises can trigger the relaxation response. It's easy to do and requires no special equipment. Sit or lie comfortably, close your eyes and breathe naturally—don't try to control your breathing. As you inhale and exhale, focus your attention on your breath and how the body moves. Notice how your chest rises and falls, and how the rib cage and stomach expand and contract. Continue to concentrate on your breath, and if random thoughts pop into your head, gently push them away and focus on your breathing again. After several minutes, this concentrated focus should result in slower, deeper breaths and a more relaxed body. You can begin with 2 or 3 minutes and gradually work up to 10–15 minutes each day. This type of breathing exercise can also be used when you're faced with a particularly stressful situation.

Meditation is similar to deep breathing, but instead of emptying your mind and concentrating only on your breath, meditation involves training your attention and awareness on something specific, while letting go of stressful thoughts. The benefits of meditation have been well known for centuries in Eastern cultures, but have only recently gained popularity in Western medicine. Like deep breathing exercises, meditation has been shown in clinical trials to produce the same physiological changes that contribute to good health (e.g., reduced heart rate and blood pressure). In addition, meditation has proven helpful in adopting other healthy lifestyle changes, such as supporting weight loss and smoking cessation, as well as reducing the symptoms of depression.

There are many types of meditative practices, including mindfulness meditation, guided meditation, transcendental meditation, yoga, and others. However, at its most basic, meditation can be practiced at home without special instruction. Begin as you would a deep breathing exercise, by sitting or lying comfortably with your eyes closed. Start to breathe in and out naturally. Once you've established a rhythm to your breathing, begin to focus your thoughts on something specific—a certain aspect of your life, such as your family, your job, or your health—or even a certain area of your body that may need healing, such as your heart. Some people prefer to focus on a phrase, repeating it silently in their head with each breath. Whatever you choose, the trick is to maintain your focus, while keeping other thoughts at bay. This is harder than it sounds. Thousands of thoughts cross our minds each day, and we are constantly receiving new stimuli. If unwanted thoughts enter your mind, simply push them aside and refocus. The goal is to put all your awareness on one thought, calming your mind and relaxing your body completely. As with anything new, meditation takes practice. Start with a few minutes a day and lengthen the time as you learn to fully concentrate. There are also many effective guided meditations available on compact disc or online, which can help you achieve better results.

Exercise When you exercise, your pituitary gland releases endorphins, which are sometimes called the "feel-good" hormones. Endorphins are really neurotransmitters that help the body relieve pain and reduce stress. You can think of them as the opposing forces to stress hormones, such as adrenaline and cortisol. Perhaps you've heard of the "runner's high," which avid runners sometimes describe as a feeling of euphoria they experience after a run? This is caused by the release of endorphins.

But you don't need to be a runner to experience stress relief. Virtually any form of exercise, from walking to yoga, can reduce stress. Studies show that physical activity not only relieves stress, it can also improve the symptoms of depression. In addition to pumping up your endorphins, exercise helps distract us from our worries and clears our heads. After a long walk or a game of tennis, you may find that you've forgotten about the pressures of the day. Muscle tension is also relieved by movement, which aids in stress relief.

Social Support There is a strong connection between relationships and stress, as well as overall health. It's important for us, as humans, to have close ties with family, friends, and other members of the community. Even pet ownership can contribute to heart health! Research shows that having a pet can lower heart rates and blood pressure, and help you feel calmer and more relaxed. This makes sense, since negative emotions can adversely affect your health, while positive emotions promote healing.

Finding time to foster good relationships and relying on those relationships for support are important for reducing stress and staying healthy. Try scheduling a regular get-together with good friends, establishing a weekly family night, or even volunteering your time to help others. These bonds are good for the heart, both figuratively and literally!

CHAPTER FOURTEEN

Heart Smart at Every Age

Everyone is the age of their heart.

UNKNOWN

During my annual physical exam, one of the questions my physician asked me was, "Have you experienced any changes in your health?" My first reaction was to say "no," but when I took a moment to think about it, I realized there were a few minor changes to report. As much we sometimes hate to admit it, it's normal to experience changes in our health as we age. Being aware of these changes and attending to them is the best way to stay healthy. Having an open and honest dialogue with your health-care provider can also go a long way toward maintaining your health.

We have long understood that cardiovascular risk increases with age, particularly for men. However, the unique aspects of a woman's biology, including pregnancy and childbirth, along with perimenopause and menopause, may also influence our risk for cardiovascular disease. Throughout our lives, the habits we adopt and the decisions we make regarding our health can have a major impact on our hearts, the quality of our life, and our longevity. Aging may be inevitable, but developing heart disease is not. As I've said before, the best treatment for heart disease, as well as other health issues, is prevention—in every stage of your life.

Young Adults (20s and 30s)

For many young women, the risk of heart disease, which is typically 40 or more years away, does not seem like a pressing issue—especially when there is so much going on! This is the age of carving your path in life, which may include completing your education, finding a job, launching a career, getting married, and starting a family. Though retirement appears distant, a good financial advisor will tell you this is the best time to start saving for the future. And, just like investing in a retirement fund, investing in your health when you're young will pay off down the road. We're all told that pennies saved now can provide for us when we're older, but we're rarely taught that healthy behaviors at this age can significantly contribute to our well-being as we age.

Recently, epidemiologists and cardiologists began looking at the *lifetime* risk for cardiovascular disease rather than the ten-year increments we had used in the past. The results of these studies are worrisome: as women, our lifetime risk of developing cardiovascular disease is increasing, mostly due to unhealthy behaviors that begin when we're young. But we can reverse those trends by making simple lifestyle changes.

Lifestyle Considerations
Diet and Exercise Younger women often lead very busy lives and, consequently, don't always think about meal preparation or exercise—especially in relation to their hearts. Yet for every year you

engage in healthy habits such as eating a good diet and exercising regularly, you reduce your lifetime risk for heart disease. It's like money in the bank! A diet high in fiber, low in sodium, and loaded with fruits and vegetables (see chapter 11) will not only help you stay fit and give you the energy you need for these busy years, it will ward off high cholesterol, diabetes, and hypertension.

Yes, even at this age, reducing sodium is important. Research has demonstrated that a diet high in sodium is not good for our bodies at any age, even as children and young adults. When you combine a high-sodium diet with weight gain, you create a recipe for the development of high blood pressure as early as your 20s or 30s. Hypertension starting in young adulthood contributes to poor vascular health, which leads to increased risk for stroke and heart disease.

This brings us to a hot topic among women of all ages: weight. Though a large number of young women say they have dieted, or are currently dieting, and retail shelves are overflowing with weight-loss aids, we have an epidemic of obesity in this country. According to the Centers for Disease Control (CDC), which monitors statistics over a number of decades, there has been a significant increase in weight or body mass index (BMI) in young adults. This trend is certainly contributing to the rise in diabetes among younger women. Increased weight also poses a greater risk for hypertension. In fact, we now understand the importance of maintaining a healthy weight starting in childhood, as it relates to many health issues. During this busy phase in your life, it's important to keep an eye on your weight—if the pounds start to sneak on, it's time to make a change. However, I will tell you what I suspect many of you already know: crash dieting, yo-yo dieting, and weight-loss gimmicks are not the answer!

Just as being overweight is not good for your heart, being too thin can also be harmful. Eating disorders are prevalent in America, particularly among young women. Anorexia and bulimia, both of which are fairly common, can be very damaging to the heart. In fact, women with extreme anorexia can die of heart failure. In addition, many restrictive or fad diets, and weight-loss aids as well, can have serious long-term health consequences. Our bodies need good fuel in the form of lean proteins, complex carbohydrates, and healthy fats in order to build muscle, repair cells, and maintain a functional vascular system. Despite the images we see in the media, the goal is not to be supermodel thin, but to keep your weight in a healthy range. Eating a balanced, nutritious diet and finding time for exercise are the best ways to achieve that objective.

I understand that finding time for exercise can be a challenge. However, regular exercise, particularly if you have a sedentary job, is critical for heart health. Even taking short breaks and getting up from your desk periodically can help. Walking during lunch is a good way to reduce stress and rev up your cardiovascular system. Personally, I think some midday exercise can boost efficiency. Here at the University of Michigan, the physiologists in our cardiac rehabilitation program use the exercise equipment during their lunch breaks, which reinforces the message to rehab patients that regular exercise is good for everyone. In addition, most of our nursing staff lace up their walking shoes at lunchtime, and many of our cardiologists are regular runners—several have completed triathlons!

It makes sense for workplaces to support healthy habits such as exercise. Employers are increasingly recognizing the benefits of offering programs and perks that contribute to keeping their employees healthy. Does your workplace offer exercise facilities of which you can take advantage? If not, perhaps you and some of your coworkers could form a walking group or exercise club? Online communities are another good resource for supporting and motivating friends and/or coworkers to get moving. Whether it's at work, at home, or at the gym, it's important to get into the habit of exercising *most* days of the week. (See chapter 12 for more exercise strategies.)

Sleep We are a sleep-deprived society. The CDC estimates that 50 to 70 million Americans have some type of sleep or wakefulness disorder, and surveys suggest the majority of our population gets less than the recommended snooze time. With so many demands on our schedule, it can be difficult to get enough sleep. When you're young, you may not feel the full effects of that sleep deprivation, but it catches up to you—in ways that may be surprising. For instance, research shows that poor sleep habits can lead to an increased appetite and therefore to overeating and obesity. This occurs because lack of sleep is associated with higher levels of gherlin, a hormone produced in the stomach and intestines that stimulates appetite.

Researchers have also linked sleep deprivation to irregular heart rhythms, such as atrial fibrillation, as well as atherosclerosis and diabetes. The deep stages of sleep are a rest period for the cardiovascular system, during which your heart rate and blood pressure fall. When you aren't getting enough of this restorative sleep, your heart is working overtime. Studies have also found that people who are chronically sleep deprived have elevated levels of C-reactive protein in their blood. As you may remember, this protein is a marker for inflammation, which contributes to atherosclerosis. So, you can see why developing good sleep habits when you're young can protect your heart over time.

Alcohol A busy social calendar often goes hand in hand with alcoholic beverages. Moderate alcohol consumption is not harmful to your heart. In fact, drinking alcohol in *moderation* has been linked to heart health due to its ability to boost HDL (good) cholesterol. But, what does moderate mean? For women, that's considered one alcoholic drink per day, which is defined as 1.5 ounces of spirits, 5 ounces of wine, or 12 ounces of beer.

Consuming too much alcohol can increase your risk for a weakened heart muscle, along with other cardiac problems, such as hypertension and atrial fibrillation. Of course, pregnant women should avoid alcohol. Also, if you are taking any medications, be sure to ask your physician about possible reactions or restrictions involving alcohol.

Smoking There is no other way to say it: smoking is bad for your health! The list of damage smoking can cause to your body, including your heart, is long (see chapter 9). If you smoke, now is the time to stop. In addition to increasing your overall cardiovascular risk, women who smoke have cardiac events such as heart attacks about 10 to 15 years earlier than women who don't smoke. Data from our medical facility have also found that women who smoke are much more likely to develop complications after having a heart attack compared to other women, and even men who smoke.

Know Your Numbers Many young women are not concerned about their cholesterol levels, blood glucose, or blood pressure, particularly if they are active and healthy. But this is the time to have all your numbers checked to determine a baseline and head off problems before they become serious. Once you know your numbers, you and your physician can keep track of trends that may occur. Understanding your personal risk factors for heart disease is the first step in prevention. If you have a family history of cardiovascular disease, diabetes, or elevated cholesterol, you should have your blood glucose and cholesterol levels checked earlier and more often.

While hypertension is more prevalent among older women, keeping tabs on your blood pressure from an early age is important. Although many women believe that 120 mmHg for the top number (systolic blood pressure) and 80 mmHg for the bottom number (diastolic blood pressure) is a good target, that's actually the *highest* reading in the normal range. If your blood pressure is even slightly higher than 120/80 mmHg, you are considered prehypertensive, which is a signal to modify your lifestyle before you require medication. Again, weight can play a key role in blood pressure control. Even a 5 to 10 pound weight gain or loss can make a significant difference in your blood pressure. A healthy weight, a diet low in sodium, not smoking, and regular exercise are central to preventing hypertension as you age.

Family Plans For many women, the 20s and 30s is prime time for thinking about or starting a family, which makes maintaining a healthy lifestyle even more important. As we discussed in previous chapters, high blood pressure and elevated blood glucose can put you and your baby at risk. Having these conditions during pregnancy can also increase your chances of developing cardiovascular disease later in life. Diet and exercise are your best weapons against the development of gestational diabetes, pre-eclampsia, and future heart problems.

If you have a history of heart disease, including congenital problems, it's very important to discuss these conditions with your physician prior to getting pregnant. Many congenital heart problems can increase the possibility of complications for both you and your baby during pregnancy. Also, if you have had postpartum cardiomyopathy (a weakened heart muscle), having another baby can be risky. In these cases, keeping in close touch with your cardiologist and other health-care providers before, during, and after pregnancy is essential.

While discussing family, I also want to emphasize that when you're healthy, your family will benefit in many ways. You don't need a doctor to tell you that a good diet, regular exercise, and proper sleep habits will give you more energy—something all parents need! But what you may not have considered is that you are the best role model for your family. The healthy habits you adopt are typically mimicked by your children. In many ways, women are the ultimate health-care providers. We are generally responsible for grocery shopping, meal preparation, first aid, scheduling check-ups, and, of course, providing commonsense advice. As such, we have a wonderful opportunity to instill healthy habits in our children that will last a lifetime.

Even if you're not planning on having a family, you can still serve as a role model for friends, relatives, and coworkers. Whether you are providing support to others or receiving support yourself, choosing to live a healthy lifestyle is easier with the help of others. Healthy behaviors can be contagious!

If you're not planning on having children, or you're postponing pregnancy, birth control is something to consider as it relates to heart health. For most women, choice of birth control will not significantly impact risk for heart disease. However, oral contraceptives can increase your chances of developing blood clots, particularly if you smoke, which can lead to stroke. Be sure to discuss your medical history and current health issues with your physician when you are considering birth control options.

A Woman in Her 20s and 30s Should:

- Invest in her health by adopting good habits, such as eating a heart-healthy diet, maintaining a healthy weight, exercising regularly, and getting proper sleep.
- Quit smoking and consume alcohol only in moderation.
- Have her cholesterol, blood glucose, and blood pressure checked regularly (every two to five years, depending on risk factors) and monitor changes. (See the sidebar on screening for more information.)
- Prepare for pregnancy by maintaining a healthy lifestyle.

The Midlife Years (40s and 50s)

A popular comedian once likened middle-aged women to taffy—constantly being pulled in many directions, but still expected to be sweet! These two decades can be extremely busy. Careers are often in full swing, demanding a great deal of time and energy. Women who are raising children have the added responsibilities of child care, school functions, sporting events, and homework sessions. A large number of women also find themselves caring for elderly parents, as well as young children. Because many women are postponing families, there can be a lot of variability during these years; while some are watching their grown children leave the nest and welcoming grandchildren, others are still immersed in child-rearing. Wherever you are in regard to career or family, taking care of your health is often a second priority at this age.

Hopefully, after reading this book, you'll understand why examining your cardiovascular health during the midlife years is so important. As we've seen, for a long time medical experts focused on the low ten-year risk that young women have for developing cardiac problems. However, in recent years a shift has occurred: we now look at the *lifetime* risk for heart disease, which for women is high. By initiating preventive measures earlier in life—keeping cholesterol low, maintaining a healthy blood pressure, and controlling chronic stress—we can reduce lifetime risk significantly. If you reach age 50 without any cardiac risk factors, your lifetime risk for cardiovascular mortality is much lower. I like to tell my patients this is the best birthday present you can give yourself! In fact, women of any age would be wise to think of low cholesterol and healthy blood pressure as valuable gifts. And, if you have one or more risk factors, such as hypertension or diabetes, then keeping them well controlled is better than jewelry!

Women are natural caregivers and are, therefore, often more focused on helping others than caring for ourselves. But taking care of yourself is vital if you plan to help others. It reminds me of the instructions flight attendants give on the plane: put your own oxygen mask on before assisting others. If you're not healthy, you won't be effective in whatever role you play in life. As importantly, if you plan to retire—perhaps do some traveling, adopt a new hobby, or enjoy your grandchildren—you need to invest in your health now to maintain vibrancy later.

Consider this: at the age of 40, a woman's lifetime risk for developing cardiovascular disease is greater than 1 out of 2. The lifetime risk for heart disease is 1 out of 3; for atrial fibrillation, it's 1 out of 4; and for both heart failure and stroke, it's 1 out of 5. What can you do to beat those odds?

Lifestyle Considerations

Diet and Exercise All the same lifestyle considerations we discussed for women in their 20s and 30s still apply. In fact, healthy habits may be even more important during these two decades as you counteract changes that occur with aging. For instance, both blood pressure and cholesterol levels tend to increase with age, so maintaining healthy ranges with diet and exercise is vital. As we've seen in previous chapters, a heart-healthy diet and regular exercise can go a long way toward preventing hypertension, high cholesterol, and diabetes.

We have talked about what it means to eat a heart-healthy diet at length, but I want to emphasize the importance of good nutrition as you age. As the threat of developing cardiac risk factors and cardiovascular disease increases, diet becomes your secret weapon. Eating a diet low in sodium is key to preventing hypertension or keeping it under control if you already have this diagnosis.

Likewise, reducing saturated fats, increasing fiber, and filling up on fruits and vegetables will keep cholesterol in a healthy range, prevent weight gain, and provide proper nutrition.

Women often gain weight during these years, and given our busy schedules, we may find it difficult to keep the extra pounds off. In addition, the hormonal changes that occur during this time can lead to stubborn weight gain. Staying active, or perhaps boosting your activity level, is more important than ever. Again, any time you can squeeze some exercise into your day is good. Even a 10–15 minute walk in the morning or at lunch, and then another 10–15 minute hike in the evening may mean the difference between maintaining a healthy weight and becoming obese. If you're trying to lose weight, you'll need to pick up the pace. Keeping your gym bag in the car, finding friends to work out with and keep you motivated, and scheduling regular times to exercise are a few strategies (see chapter 12 for more).

Besides maintaining a healthy weight, exercise at this age is necessary to prevent the loss of muscle mass and keep bones strong. As we age, all of us lose lean muscle mass and gain fat mass, which means that even if you don't gain weight, you may have more fat than is good for you. Women tend to gain weight around the waist, particularly during the perimenopausal years. In addition to being frustrating, this type of weight gain is unhealthy. An expanding waistline often signals an increase in visceral adiposity, a type of fat that impacts cardiovascular health. Visceral adiposity is also associated with poor glucose control, which leads to diabetes, elevated blood pressure, and poor vascular health.

If your weight is not in a healthy range or your activity level is low, this is the age to make some changes. It's never too late to start eating a heart-healthy diet and exercising five or more days a week. Remember, 80 percent of heart disease risk is modifiable with lifestyle changes.

Know Your Numbers Women in their 40s and 50s need to know their numbers. What is your blood pressure? Has it been creeping upward? What is your cholesterol profile? Are you seeing an increase in LDL (bad) cholesterol and a decrease in HDL (good) cholesterol? What is your fasting glucose level? If you don't know the answers to these questions, it's time to schedule a physical exam! If you know your numbers, you can compare them with levels that are considered optimal for women your age using many online resources (see Resources). As you age, you should be diligent about checking these numbers periodically and keeping track of any changes. If your numbers are moving in the wrong direction, you can work with your physician to reverse these trends.

Perimenopause and Menopause Entering the menopausal years can be very challenging for many women. Changes in estrogen and progesterone are signs that the body is moving out of the reproductive years. Though natural, these hormonal changes can cause a wide range of uncomfortable symptoms. During perimenopause, hot flashes and night sweats are very common. These vasomotor symptoms typically increase in the final year prior to the last menstrual period and during the first year of menopause. However, some women may continue to experience these problems for years, even decades. Finding relief can be important, not only because these symptoms interfere with daily activities, but also because they interrupt sleep cycles.

Unfortunately, despite numerous studies on various treatments, there is no magic solution. Several trials of natural supplements, including black cohosh and soy, have been conducted with mixed success; they may work for some women, but not for others. Quite honestly, researchers don't really understand how to alleviate these symptoms for the majority of women, other than hormone replacement therapy (HRT).

As part of the Women's Health Initiative (WHI) and other large-scale studies, researchers found that HRT does appear to reduce or eliminate hot flashes and night sweats for most women. However, there are risks related to HRT. For women with heart disease, HRT can increase the chances for future cardiac events. In addition, we now know that HRT does not appear to benefit postmenopausal women in the prevention of heart disease. This is an important revelation. During my training, we encouraged postmenopausal women to use HRT in order to lower their cholesterol. Based on observations, we thought HRT reduced a woman's cardiovascular risk. It was only after larger, controlled studies were conducted that we found no related benefit. In fact, in the WHI study, the risk for heart attacks and stroke actually *increased* with HRT. Hormone replacement therapy also increased the risk for blood clots in women's legs (which can be very dangerous if a clot travels to the lungs), as well as breast cancer.

Many questions remain about HRT, and the results are by no means definitive. First of all, these trials used predominantly one type of pill, which means we do not know the risks or benefits associated with other types of HRT. Unfortunately, because these large trials cost millions of dollars, it's unlikely that studies of this type and scale will be conducted in the near future. As of now, for women who do not have heart disease, the question of taking a hormone replacement to reduce hot flashes should be discussed thoroughly with their health-care provider. It's important to ask your physician how HRT impacts your personal risk for heart disease, based on your past medical history and current health status. These discussions should include the types of HRT available and the duration of use. Be sure to let your physician know about any vitamins or supplements you may be taking, as these can affect HRT.

- Maintain a heart-healthy diet and exercise regularly (at least 30 minutes on five or more days each week). In particular, sodium intake should be less than 2,000 mg per day to counteract natural increases in blood pressure.
- Know her numbers—have cholesterol, blood pressure, and blood glucose levels checked every one to five years, depending on risk factors.
- Consider medication, in conjunction with lifestyle changes, to keep high cholesterol, prediabetes, and prehypertension in check.
- Continue taking prescribed medications, as directed, if they have been diagnosed with cardiac risk factors.

The Senior Years (60s, 70s, and Beyond)

Today's seniors are more active than ever. I am always inspired by women in their 60s, 70s, and beyond who are embarking on second careers, adopting new hobbies, taking on volunteer work, and checking off items on their bucket list. Compared to earlier generations, the possibilities for women in this age group are expansive. Seniors account for a large and growing portion of our population, which means there are examples of healthy aging all around us. Unfortunately, it also means there are more people with cardiovascular problems.

The majority of women who experience heart attacks and strokes do so during this stage of life (age 60 and older). When it comes to cardiovascular risk, women typically lag about ten years behind men—a man's risk increases in his 50s, while a woman's risk becomes greater in her 60s. Although they are common, developing cardiac problems as we age is not a given. As we've learned, a vast majority of cardiovascular issues can be prevented. In fact, I sometimes see women in their 80s and 90s who are healthier and more active than women half their age, due to their lifestyle choices. So, what's the secret to healthy aging?

The way we age can vary greatly. Our genes form part of the picture, but they do not tell the entire story. While we don't have therapies to change our genetic makeup, we can control the environmental factors that influence aging. As I said earlier, I think of these factors as an investment for retirement. Even if you haven't invested wisely in your health up to now, you can still reduce your cardiovascular risks by adopting a healthy lifestyle in your senior years. It's never too late to become heart smart.

Lifestyle Considerations

Diet and Exercise It's not surprising that the same heart-healthy diet recommendations outlined for younger women still apply and may be even more important as we age. Since hypertension is very common among older women, reducing sodium intake even further is essential. In addition, cholesterol levels tend to rise with age, so reducing saturated fats and increasing fiber are vital to maintaining a healthy cholesterol profile.

Social isolation can often have a negative influence on eating well at this age. Empty nesters and those who have lost a spouse often find it difficult to cook healthy meals for one (or even two). Many of my older patients tell me they find themselves snacking or relying on packaged meals rather than cooking. It's important to make the effort to prepare healthy, well-balanced meals. Try preparing larger meals and freezing portions for later, or partnering with others to make several meals at once. Instead of a book club, why not form a cooking club? Not only can you improve your diet by focusing on low-sodium and high-fiber recipes, but you'll also benefit from the social aspect!

Social connections can also help you get regular exercise. While many of us see exercise as a chore, it can be an enjoyable part of your routine when done with a partner who keeps you motivated. And exercise is very important as you age. As the saying goes, "if you don't use it, you lose it." Muscle mass is lost naturally through the aging process, so staying active is necessary to retain lean muscle, reduce fat, and keep our bones strong. In addition, muscles help your body process glucose more efficiently, which prevents diabetes.

Another important consideration as you get older is your ability to maintain balance and strength, which can help you prevent falls. I always worry about women who have been injured by a fall or are fearful of falling, as they are more likely to reduce their activities. By becoming sedentary, they are not only less fit and more prone to falling, but they also increase their risk for heart disease.

For many older women, the opportunity for regular exercise was not available when they were younger. Exercise was getting the housework done! In today's more automated world, this type of work is not as strenuous and doesn't provide enough exercise to keep fit. We also have less work to do as children get older and move away. This means that many older women become more sedentary without even realizing it—which makes this the perfect time to explore new activities. Taking daily walks with a friend, joining a swim group or water aerobics class, or learning the gentle movements of tai chi can keep you moving in ways to which you look forward. Most communities have recreational facilities geared toward seniors, which are great places to discover new interests and new friends.

When I emphasize the importance of staying functionally active, some of my older patients express frustration with arthritis and other impairments that limit their activities. It's true that you may not be able to do the same activities you once did, but there is always something you can do. Start by asking your doctor for suggestions, or consult with a physical therapist. You can also check out community resources. Because our population is aging, the number of specialized programs for seniors has increased dramatically. Low-impact yoga, water aerobics, and exercise equipment designed specifically for older adults are just a few of the options available. If you are no longer able to drive, ask about free transportation services for seniors offered by many communities.

If you have had a heart attack or stroke, you can still benefit from regular exercise. Even patients with significant cardiac problems such as heart failure can improve their quality of life by staying active. Be sure to ask your physician what types of activities you can safely do. Many cardiac rehabilitation centers will let patients continue to exercise at their facilities after the program is completed (e.g., after a heart attack). Personally, I know many women who have continued to go to rehab for years—enjoying not only the exercise, but also the people they meet.

Social Connections You may have noticed the focus on group activities. That's because social support is good for your heart! Studies show that social isolation can not only increase your risk for heart disease, but also elevate your chances for future cardiac problems after you've had a heart attack or stroke. It may be that women have a hard time maintaining a healthy lifestyle without the support of others. Certainly, if those around you are supportive, you are more likely to stick to good behaviors such as exercise. Having the support of friends or family may also reduce stress and keep depression at bay, which contribute to heart health.

Sadly, older women are more likely to be widowed or have limited access to meeting others, which makes social isolation more prevalent in this group. If you find yourself in this situation, it's important to get out and remain social. Again, senior centers are a good resource for meeting others, learning new hobbies, and staying active, as well as providing transportation to those who are homebound.

Take as Directed It's very common for women in this age group to take medication to help control cardiac risk factors such as hypertension and high cholesterol. However, medication is not a miracle cure! A healthy diet and regular physical activity can reduce the need to increase dosages and make your medications work more effectively. For example, many women with hypertension require two or three medications to regulate their blood pressure, particularly older women with a long history of hypertension. However, some patients need to take four or five medications to do the same job. I often wonder whether, if these women were able to modify their lifestyle—reduce sodium intake, increase activity, or lose weight—would they still require the additional medications?

If you are using medications, it's important to take them as directed. The number of patients who forget to take their medications is staggering! Skipping doses or even taking them at different times of the day can lead to problems. Using a pill box with compartments for each day of the week, keeping medications handy (i.e., in your purse, on the counter, next to your toothbrush), and setting an alarm on your phone are a few ways to make sure you stay on track. Even a simple note taped to the refrigerator or the bathroom mirror is a good reminder.

You should also keep in mind that as we age, our metabolism slows down, which means our bodies don't metabolize or process substances like alcohol efficiently. As a result, you may find that you have to limit or, in some cases, avoid alcohol, particularly if you are taking medications. Be sure to check labels or consult with your physician/pharmacist about any possible interactions.

Comfort for Caregivers Many women in this age group are caring for partners who are ill. Caregiver stress is very prevalent in today's society. In addition to the chronic stress associated with taking care of a loved one, caregivers often neglect their own health, including not eating right or exercising, as well as skipping regular checkups. In order to be effective, it's important for caregivers to set aside time for their own care. Stress reduction should be a top priority—even a few minutes of deep breathing or other relaxation techniques throughout the day are beneficial. Activities such as brisk walking, broken up into 10 minute periods, can also alleviate stress while keeping you fit. Remember, studies from the Harvard Nurses' Health Study demonstrated that brisk walking in 10 minute intervals can reduce the risk for heart disease. If you take three of these breaks each day, you'll be getting the recommended level of activity for heart health. Getting help with tasks is also important. Taking a break will not only improve your mental health, it's also good for your heart.

Know Your Numbers I am always surprised (and a bit dismayed) to find that many women stop scheduling annual physical exams as they get older. While it's true that some tests are not required annually after the reproductive years, a general exam that includes a blood pressure reading, cholesterol profile, blood glucose test, and questions regarding overall health is absolutely necessary. If you have been diagnosed with a risk factor such as hypertension or diabetes, then regular checkups are important to monitor the condition and reassess medications. It's always better to catch a potential problem in the early stages than to wait until it becomes more serious. Developing a trusting and open relationship with your health-care provider is an important part of aging well.

A Woman in Her 60s, 70s, and Beyond Should:

- Continue following a heart-healthy diet and exercising regularly.
- Reduce sodium intake to less than 2,000 mg per day (<1,500 mg if you can!), particularly if she has been diagnosed with hypertension.
- Maintain social connections.
- Have cholesterol, blood pressure, and blood glucose levels checked every two to five years, depending on risk factors. If these numbers are elevated, tests should be performed more frequently.
- Take all medications as directed.

Screening Guidelines from the American Heart Association

Recommended Screening	How Often?	Starting When?
Cholesterol	Every 5 years for normal risk people. More often if any of the following apply to you: • Total cholesterol >200 mg/dL • Woman over age 50 or man over age 45 • HDL <50mg/dL (woman) or HDL <40mg/dL (man) • Other risk factors for coronary heart disease and stroke	Age 20
Blood pressure	Each regular health-care visit or at least once every 2 years (if blood pressure less than 120/80 mmHg)	Age 20
Blood glucose test	Every 3 years	Age 45
Weight, BMI	Each regular health-care visit	Age 20
Waist circumference	As needed to help evaluate cardiovascular risk	Age 20
Discuss smoking, physical activity & diet	Each regular health-care visit	Age 20

Getting Answers

Developing a good relationship with your physician—one that includes honest, open communications—is an essential part of a heart-healthy lifestyle. The following questions can help you make the most of your annual checkup. And, because communication is a two-way street, I've included a list of questions that your physician should be asking you.

What Every Woman Should Ask Her Physician

1. What is my overall risk for heart disease; what do I need to monitor as I age?
2. What is my blood pressure? And what is a good goal for me?
3. How can I maintain a good blood pressure?
4. What are my cholesterol numbers (including LDL, HDL, and triglycerides)? And, what is a good goal for me?
5. How can I maintain a healthy cholesterol profile as I age?
6. What is my fasting glucose and HgA1c? Am I at risk for diabetes?

7. What are my weight, body mass index (BMI), and waist circumference? Am I at goal for these numbers?
8. What can I do in terms of diet, activity, and stress management to help maintain a good cholesterol level and blood pressure?
   a. What is a good level of physical activity for me?
   b. What type of diet should I follow (i.e., low-sodium, high-fiber, low-cholesterol)?
9. Do I need medication to control my cholesterol, blood sugar, and/or blood pressure? If so, how long do I need the medication(s):
   a. Ask about duration
   b. Ask about different types of medications
   c. Ask about potential side effects (but remember, while side effects do happen often, medications effect everyone differently and may require some trial and error)
10. If you are on a special diet or are taking supplements or treatments your doctor did not prescribe, remember to ask about potential interactions with new medications.
11. How often should I review my risk factors and overall risk for heart disease?
12. Do I need special testing to assess my risk for heart disease?

Questions Women Diagnosed with Heart Disease or Other Heart Conditions Should Ask Their Physicians

1. Review your heart history. Make sure you understand what your problem entailed, including the cause, as well as what treatments you had.
2. What type of follow-up appointments do I need and how often?
3. Do I need cardiac rehabilitation?

4. What activities should I avoid, and what type of exercise is right for me?
5. What type of diet should I follow?
6. What can I do to prevent future heart events (e.g., lower blood pressure, improve cholesterol profile, keep blood sugar in a healthy range, increase activity)?

What Your Physician Should Ask You

1. Do you have a family history of premature heart disease?
2. Do you or another member of your family have a history of elevated cholesterol, hypertension, or diabetes?
3. Have you altered your exercise habits or daily activity in the past several months or years due to fatigue, shortness of breath, or other reasons?
4. A full review of symptoms is typical at initial visits. However, if you have a follow-up visit or a visit for another reason (e.g., a sore throat), your physician should ask about any changes in your health status—a new diagnosis or hospitalization, chest pain, extreme fatigue, swelling in your ankles or feet, or dizziness (see chapters 2 and 4 for a complete list of cardiac warning signs).
5. What are your current exercise habits, including the type of activity, how often, and at what intensity?
6. What are the stressors in your life? And how do you manage your stress?
7. Describe your eating habits, including how often you eat out and the amount of packaged or premade food you eat.
8. Do you smoke?
   a. If so, have you tried to quit?
   b. If you've tried quitting without success, what worked and what didn't?

c. How can I help you try to quit again (or for the first time)?

9. How many hours of sleep do you get each night?
   a. Do you snore?
   b. Do you feel tired during the day?

10. If you have ever been pregnant, were there any problems with the pregnancy?
    a. Did you have elevated blood sugar while pregnant (gestational diabetes)?
    b. Did you have high blood pressure while pregnant?
    c. What did your babies weigh at birth?

APPENDIX B

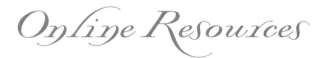

Online Resources

General References (which also have information on specific conditions and risk factors)
- HeartHealthyWomen.org
  www.hearthealthywomen.org/index.php
- American Heart Association
  *www.goredforwomen.org/about_heart_disease_*
  and_stroke.aspx
- American College of Cardiology
  www.cardiosmart.org/
- Women Heart: The National Coalition for Women with
  Heart Disease
  www.womenheart.org/

References from Chapter 5, "Assessing Your Risk"
Framingham Risk Scores To learn more about these tools, you
can visit the Framingham Study site. There are several risk

calculators, including the original ten-year risk score, the risk score for both heart disease and stroke, and a 30-year risk score.

- The Framingham Risk Score
  www.framinghamheartstudy.org/risk/coronary.html
- The General Cardiovascular Disease Risk Score
  www.framinghamheartstudy.org/risk/gencardio.html
- The Cardiovascular Disease Risk Score—30-year risk
  www.framinghamheartstudy.org/risk/cardiovascular30.html

You can also go to the National Institutes of Health, which has the Framingham 10-year Risk Score. To calculate your personal risk score, go to the online Framingham calculator: http://hp2010.nhlbihin.net/atpiii/calculator.asp

Reynolds Risk Score The web site for the Reynolds Risk Score is *www.reynoldsriskscore.org*

References from Chapter 7, "The Cholesterol Connection"

- For more information on LDL targets for patients with other risk factors, go to *www.nhlbi.nih.gov/guidelines/cholesterol/atglance.htm*
  - For more information on when to get tested, visit *www.heart.org/HEARTORG/Conditions/Cholesterol/SymptomsDiagnosisMonitoringofHighCholesterol/How-To-Get-Your-Cholesterol-Tested_UCM_305595_Article.jsp*

References from Chapter 8, "Diabetes and Your Heart"

- American Diabetes Association: *www.diabetes.org/*
  - The American Heart Association and the American College of Cardiology also provide information on diabetes as it relates to heart disease.

The American Heart Association: *www.heart.org*
The American College of Cardiology: *www.acc.com*

References from Chapter 9, "Smoke-Free for Life"

- To help parents start a dialogue regarding the dangers of smoking and to provide teens with information on smoking in a language they understand, visit www.kidshealth.org.
  - To help you quit smoking, visit web sites such as *www.smokefree.gov* and the American Lung Association's *www.lung.org/stop-smoking*, which provide advice, support, and step-by-step guidelines. Tech-savvy women can find free mobile apps such as QuitGuide to help you stay on track.

References from Chapter 11, "Eating for Life"

- For general information on heart-healthy eating, visit the American Heart Association web site at www.heart.org or the American College of Cardiology at *www.acc.com* for their CardioSmart eating guide.
- For more on the DASH diet, visit *www.dashdiet.org/*
- For more information on alternative therapies, including vitamins and supplements:
  - The National Institutes of Health has a special section called the National Center for Complementary and Alternative Medicine (NCCAM), which examines alternative therapies.
    www.nccam.nih.gov/health/supplements
    www.nccam.nih.gov/ (for information on other treatments beyond supplements)
  - The Natural Standard health web site provides high-quality, evidence-based information about complementary and alternative therapies, including

herbs and supplements: www.naturalstandard.com/
- Mayo Integrative Medicine: *www.mayoclinic.org/general-internal-medicine-rst/ cimc.html*
- Harvard: *www.brighamandwomens.org/research/osher/*

References from Chapter 12, "Get Moving"

Heart rate calculators: You can find heart rate calculators on many web sites, including *www.mayoclinic.com* and *www.active.com.*

Index

911, when to call, 34, 40, 65

Ablation, 48
ACE inhibitors, 58, 89
African-Americans, 85, 108
Age, as a risk factor
  in gestational diabetes, 120, 122
  in heart disease, 66, 68, 70
  in high blood pressure, 85
  in high cholesterol, 94
Aging and health
  in midlife, 196–201
  in the senior years, 201–7
  for young adults, 189–95
Alcohol
  binge drinking and AFib, 46, 193
  contributing to high blood pressure, 85
  guidelines for consuming, 156
  stress leading to use of, 181
  SVT caused by, 49
  use by young adults, 192–93
American Cancer Society, 132
American Diabetes Association (ADA), 114, 122
American Heart Association
  on changing behaviors, 140
  on cholesterol, 93, 103
  dietary recommendations of, 144, 147
  on exercise, 168, 170
  heart attack warning signs from, 34
  on smoking, 127
  for smoking cessation information, 132
  statistics on cardiovascular diseases, 26
  statistics on gender, diabetes and
    heart disease, 109
  web site, 21, 170
American Institute in Medicine, on fiber, 152
American Lung Association, 131, 132
Angina, 30–31, 57
Anorexia, 191
Anti-depressants, 58
Anxiety, as symptom of heart attack, 33, 54
Aorta, 16, 18, 19–20
Arrhythmias
  atrial fibrillation ("AFib"), 45–49
  bradycardia, 44, 45, 50
  diagnosing, 51
  overview of, 22, 43–44
  pacemakers for, 50
  sudden cardiac death caused by, 61–62
  supraventricular (SVT), 49
  tachycardia, 45, 51
  types of, 44
Arteries, 19, 77–78, 112, 125–26
Arterioles, 78
Asians, 119
Aspirin, 35, 47, 55–56
Atherosclerosis
  angina and, 31
  diabetes contributing to, 112
  heart attacks resulting from, 29
  LDL cholesterol impact on, 101, 103
  as leading cause of heart disease, 23, 27
  overview of, 23, 26
  preventive measures for, 42
  problems related to, 18
  role of in heart health, 19–20, 28

role of in strokes, 38
smoking contributing to, 126
Atria, 15, 16, 17
Atrial fibrillation ("AFib"), 45–46, 47, 48–49
Autoimmune conditions, 110
Automatic external defibrillators (AEDs), 22

Benson, Herbert, 184
Beta-blockers, 58, 59, 61, 89
Birth control, 96, 127, 197
Blood glucose level, 72, 96, 119, 165, 207
  See also Diabetes
Blood pressure
  See also High blood pressure
  classification of, 82
  exercise as benefit to, 165
  fluctuation of, 82–83
  follow-up recommendations, 84
  know your numbers, 81–84
  low, 89–90
  in metabolic syndrome, 119
  overview of, 77
  prehypertension, 82–84
  in risk assessment, 72
  weight and, 84–85, 194
Body mass index (BMI), 70, 72, 159, 190, 207
Bradycardia, 44, 45, 50
Broken heart syndrome, 60–61, 180–81
Bulimia, 191
Bupropion, 131–32
Bypass surgery, 36

Caffeine, 51
Calcium channel blockers, 59, 89
Cancer, deaths from compared to
  heart disease, 26, 52
Capillaries, 78
Cardiac catheterization, 35–36
Cardiac MRI, 57
Cardiac rehabilitation, 37–38, 169, 204
Cardiovascular disease, 26, 39
  See also Heart Disease; Strokes
Caregiver stress, 206
Centers for Disease Control and
  Prevention, 127–28, 170, 190, 192
Chambers of the heart, 17
Change, stages of, 137–40
Chest pain
  causes of, 30–31, 32
  heart attack risk increased by, 56
  as warning sign, 54
  in women, 32–33
Children
  fish restrictions for, 147
  impact of secondhand smoke on, 130
  including in exercise activities, 172, 173, 174
  meal planning and preparation participation
    by, 161, 162
  online resources for, 129
Cholesterol
  See also High-density lipoproteins (HDL)
    (good cholesterol); Low-density lipoproteins
    (LDL) (bad cholesterol)
  affect of exercise on, 107
  affects on the heart, 98
  anabolic steroids affecting, 101

217

Acknowledgments

There are numerous people who have helped me along my path in medicine. Without my parents and my Tanta Clista, who never wavered in their determination to convince me I can do anything if I put my mind to it, I would not have gone back to school to complete premed course work and apply for medical school. Their belief in my abilities, despite my being dyslexic, made me believe that I, too, could be successful academically. My teachers at Milton Academy, in particular Mrs. Daily, supported me on my path from a less than stellar student to a doctor. These educators supported their students, demanding that they grow and become passionate, curious members of society. Physicians are educators as well; I can only hope that I will inspire my patients and providers in training as I was inspired by my parents and teachers.

I want to acknowledge and thank those colleagues with whom I have worked, both past and present. My administrative assistant Cindy Harper, who is my peripheral brain, supporter, and friend. She is the glue of my workplace life—without whom this book would not have been written. I also want to thank my colleagues who provide a supportive and happy place to work. Dr. Kim Eagle was one of the first cardiologists I met from the University of Michigan, more than 10 years ago; he always has time to talk and support those around him. Dr. David Pinsky, Linda Larin, and the other Cardiovascular Directors have sustained my academic pursuits and passions—I thank them for their support. Thank you to my mentors, Drs. Emelia Benjamin, Caroline Richardson, and Sioban Harlow, who have promoted my love of prevention and women's health. Marilyn Cramer and the members of the pre-award grants administration; Marilyn is a cheerleader extra-ordinaire for all of us working on advancing clinical research. Thank you also to the members of the Women's Heart Program who have a deep dedication to women's health.

When embarking on this book, I was not sure how the whole process would evolve. Without the help of Lynne Johnson, my editor, I would not have known where to begin. She also was encouraging and accessible. In particular I want to thank Robin Porter, writer extraordinaire who went through every chapter with diligence and expertise. Her skillful writing allows my voice to come through without the spelling and grammatical errors. She and Lynne answered my numerous questions about the processes and essentially took the book to higher levels. I cannot thank them enough.

Most of all, I want to thank my sons, Anders and Aric. I always say we are a team, but they translate those words into action. Without them pitching in to make dinner or do the laundry, I would not have time to get everything done in my life. They make me laugh and laughter is truly the best medicine. And I wish to thank friends around me whom I know I can always call if I need to—Caroline, Patty, and Jackie, in particular— thank you, your open hearts and homes mean so much.

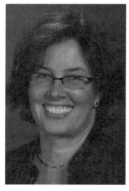

Elizabeth "Lisa" A. Jackson, MD, MPH, received her medical degree from Tufts University School of Medicine. She completed her residency in internal medicine at Brown University's Rhode Island Hospital and attended the New England Medical Center in Boston, Massachusetts, for a fellowship in cardiovascular medicine. She also completed a research fellowship in preventative medicine at the Brigham and Women's Hospital in Boston, Massachusetts. It was during her research fellowship that Dr. Jackson earned a Master's in Public Health at Harvard University's School of Public Health, where she also completed training in nutritional epidemiology.

Dr. Jackson began work at the University of Michigan Health Center in 2007. She works as an attending cardiologist with an emphasis in women's cardiovascular health and cardiovascular prevention. Dr. Jackson is board certified in Internal Medicine and Cardiovascular Disease and is a fellow of the American College of Cardiology.

Robin Porter With a background in corporate communications, Robin Porter is a versatile freelance writer, who has written a wide variety of materials. Most notably, she has authored several company history/anniversary books, as well as co-authored books on various medical issues. Robin lives with her husband, Alan, and son, Sean, in Canton, Michigan.